# REIKI

# REIKI
## A Unique Art of Healing

SUKHDEEPAK MALVAI

GYAN PUBLISHING HOUSE
NEW DELHI - 110002

**REIKI :**
A Unique Art of Healing
*(Health)*

ISBN : 81-212-0610-3



Published in 1998 in India by
Gyan Publishing House
5, Ansari Road
New Delhi 110 002
Laser Typesetting : Grow Computers, Delhi.
Printed at Mehra Offset Press, New Delhi.

*To*
*All the staff and assistants at Landmark Education,*
*who are engaged in the work of transformation*

# CONTENTS

# Preface

Reiki is a system in which hands are used as healing instruments. Due to the growing number of happy and cured patients all over the country Reiki is entering the healers, or doctors handbook. Besides taking care of physical problems, Reiki is finding wide application as a tool for personal and spiritual growth too. Reiki is able to make you whole and complete, and above all it can make you live in abundance forever. Reiki healing works on our *Aura* or bioenergy body (which permeates the physical body and extends a few inches beyond it) and *Chakras* of our body (there are seven major *chakras,* each related to an endocrinc gland). Before entering our physical body, the disease forces its way into our *aura.* Reiki healing works on the *aura* level and corrects the blocked or malfunctioning *chakras* to cure the disease. Reiki roots out the cause of the disease and there is no danger of overdose and many do's *and* don'ts. For example, in *pranic* healing, liquor, tobacco and non-vegetarian food items are believed to deplete energy and bring disharmony to the *chakras,* and sometimes the healer ends up giving excess of energy, potentially harmful for the sufferer. Reiki is getting so popular that its teaching has become a remarkably lucrative career option. Belief in Reiki is not required for Reiki to work, the principles of healing are always the same and they are not dependent upon anyone's beliefs.

I sincerely hope that this book would broaden your knowledge and open many new doors in life for you.

**Author**

# THE SYMBOL

*Reiki* written in a manner commonly used by the Reiki Alliance

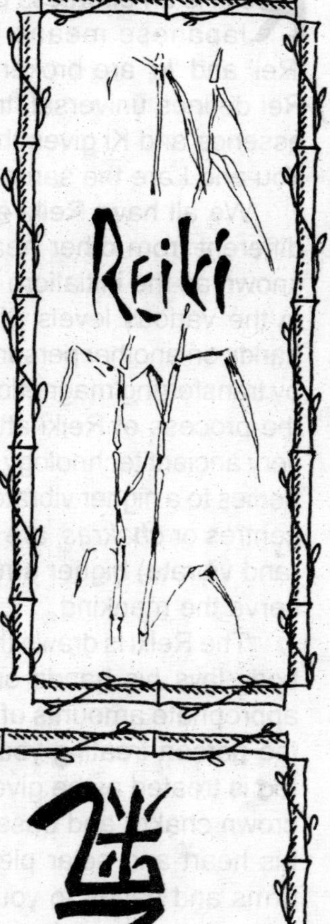


*Reiki* written in Japanese in different styles of writing

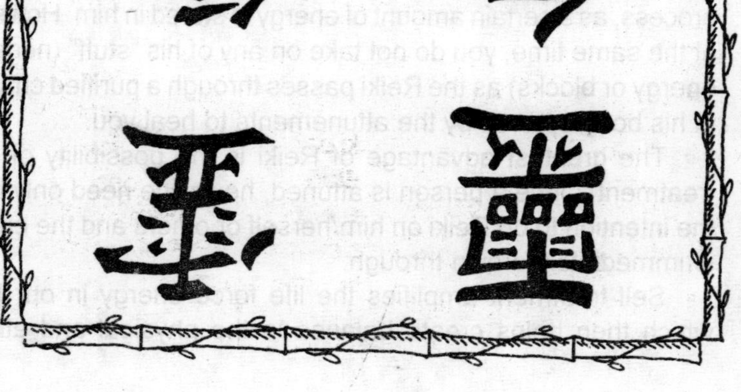

# WHAT IS REIKI ?

Reiki is an effortless process for natural healing. The Reiki in Japanese means Universal Life Force Energy. When 'Rei' and 'ki' are broken down into their two component parts, Rei defines universal, transcendental spirit, mysterious power, essence and Ki gives the meaning of the vital life force energy. You and I are the same Universal Life Force Energy.

We all have Reiki energy in ourselves. What makes Reiki different from other healing methods, is the attunement (also known as the initiation) process which the student experiences in the various levels of Reiki teachings. Anyone can lay their hands on another person and help accelerate the healing process by transferring magnetic energy. A person who has been through the process of Reiki attunements however, has experienced a very ancient technology for fine tuning of the physical and etheric bodies to a higher vibratory level. In addition, certain of the energy centres or *chakras,* are opened to enable the person to channel (and vibrate) higher amounts of Universal Life Force Energy to serve the mankind.

The Reiki is drawn through the channel. For example, if some body lays his hands on you to do a treatment, you will draw appropriate amounts of energy to areas of your body needing it, the person treating you is never drained in the process, as he too is treated as he gives a treatment. The energy enters at his crown chakra and passes through the upper energy centres to his heart and solar plexus. The rest then passes through his arms and hands to your body. He is thus never drained in the process, as a certain amount of energy is stored in him. However, at the same time, you do not take on any of his "stuff" (negative energy or blocks) as the Reiki passes through a purified channel in his body-opened by the attunements to heal you.

The greatest advantage of Reiki is the possibility of self-treatment. Once a person is attuned, he or she need only have the intention to do Reiki on him/herself or others and the energy is immediately drawn through.

Self-treatment amplifies the life force energy in our body which then helps create balance in the physical and etheric bodies. Treating oneself also helps to release withheld emotions and energy blocks. It is also a useful technique to get rid of stressful condition.

Reiki is a very ancient science hidden since many centuries, until D. Usui rediscovered this very old "technology" hidden in the Tibetan Sutras. Researchers used highly sensitive instruments which measure the flow of energy forces entering the body. They confirmed that Reiki energy enters the healer through the top of the head and exits through the hands. The energy force comes from a northerly direction, but it comes from the south when below the equator. In addition, once the Reiki energy is activated, it seems to flow in a counter clock-wise spiral motion.

The volume of energy emanating from the hands definitely increases during treatment. A well-known researcher who has developed an ingenious technique for doing life-energy interpretations with Kirlian photography, tested a Reiki master before and during the sending of an absentee healing. The photograph taken during the absentee healing displayed a marked increase of radiation when compared with the photo taken before the treatment, which had displayed a smaller range of emanations.

This indicates very clearly that there is a release of energy through the bodily system, when blocks are released. All outcomes are different for every treatment, the healee being the determining factor in the net result. Each person draws in just the right amount of life force that he or she needs to release, activate, or transform the energy of the physical and etheric bodies. Reiki not only can effect change in the chemical structure of the body, by helping to regenerate organs and rebuild tissue and bone, it also helps create balance on the mental level. Reiki is not a belief system, hence no mental preparation or direction is needed to receive a treatment, only a desire to receive and accept the energy. On the other hand, from the standpoint of the person practising Reiki, since it is not a belief system, once the intention is clear to start a treatment, it will always be activated when used as instructed. Reiki is truly a spiritual discipline, as realizing the importance of taking responsibility for all that one creates in life is indeed one of the key of Reiki.

Reiki is a wonderful tool to help one develop conscious awareness, the very key to enlightenment. As in most things in life, Reiki must be experienced to be appreciated. Reiki may surely help each individual find harmony and balance in body, spirit and mind. The exhilaration which can be experienced at each stage of awareness is unveiled gradually and makes it all worthwhile.

# HOW REIKI WORKS?

You would be curious to know how Reiki works and what it feels like to both practitioner and patient.

Each person reacts in a different way to Reiki. Since it works where the recipient need it most, no general rule can be said to exist. Some recipients of Reiki admitted that they had never experienced such a deep sense of relaxation in their whole life and some said that they were filled with a feeling of peace and quiet. A gentleman said that his legs prickled all the time and he got very restless. A lady saw many images, wonderful landscapes and colours. The most common thing experienced during treatment is a sense of peace and relaxation, often combined with a pleasant feeling of security and of being enclosed in a fine sheath of energy. But even this won't be experienced every time.

Reiki treatment is done by laying hands gently on the various parts of the body with fingers closed tight. The recipient soon feels a kind of flowing sensation, often combined with a sensation of warmth, which can turn into heat or become quite cold. The patient will often feel the flowing as noticeably as practitioners do, as well as the sensation of hot and cold. On some occasions, he will also sense warmth at a different part of the body than where we feel it, or what he experiences as warmth is cold for us.

But, if a thermometer is placed between the practitioner's hands and the patient's body it will not register a noticeable change in temperature. Obviously, the change that is experienced as taking place, cannot be measured physically.

Many Reiki recipients fall asleep during treatment, but this won't make any difference in the effects of treatment. On other occasions, old and unresolved experiences may become conscious again. A release of emotions can occur and tears will flow or a laugh of relief will be released. It has also been known for experiences of a strongly visual character to occur; this may take on a visionary character in the case of people who regularly practise a form of meditation. It can also occur that a series of treatment will bring about dissolution of inner barriers which had been blocking holistic growth in a person.

When a healer lays hands on the patient's body in order to link him to the energy of Reiki, it won't merely affect him on the material plane but will involve him in his entirety of spirit, body and mind. Physical illness or weakness is only the bodily expression of lack of basic order, a sign of having fallen out of a state of inner union with all life.

Reiki will bring you a decisive step closer to an original state of order. Reiki energy cannot be explained along the usual lines of therapeutic thinking. When someone is treated with Reiki, he is brought back into a state of unity with the harmony of the universe. This harmony, which is able to reach him in his smallest of cells, makes him whole and healthy again, the patient can heal himself by utilizing his natural ability.

Reiki opens new doors for us, it leads us to a state of wholeness. It frequently happens that patients will come into contact with new ideas after a few Reiki treatments. Some people start to meditate or practise some other kind of spiritual method. Others will change their eating habits or their approach towards life or even try to become Reiki practitioners themselves. Some patients will become aware of problems that had been repressed all along and find solutions for them. It is not seldom that a person will take certain bold and new steps or develop the wish to change something in his life. A patient should follow these positive impulses for his own good.

If one starts Reiki he will notice that the effects of treatment may differ from what he had been expecting.

Reiki has its own way or formula, knowing where and to what extent it is required. For this reason, it is not necessary to make a diagnosis before treatment, a fact that spares us no few mistakes. Every now and then patients come with certain complaints only to discover after treatment that other things have helped him a lot which looked insignificant in the beginning.

## THE MAIN FEATURES OF REIKI

- **REIKI** strengthens both body and soul.
- **REIKI** re-establishes spiritual equilibrium and mental well being.

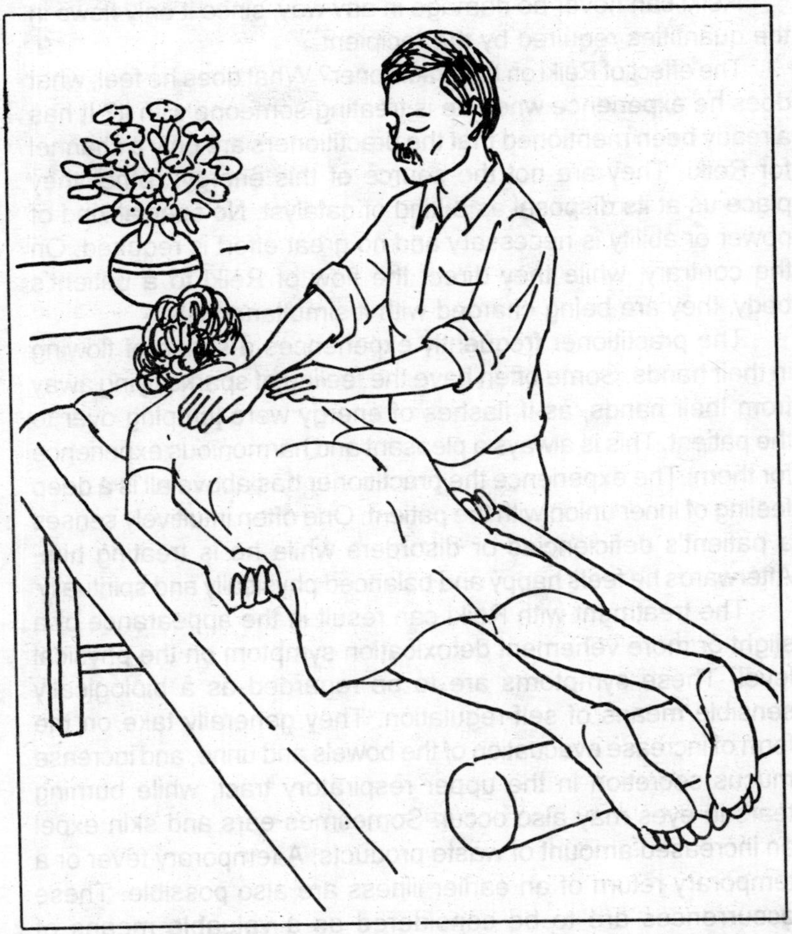

- **REIKI** functions on all levels, whether mental or spiritual, physical or emotional.
- **REIKI** encourages the body's natural ability to heal itself.
- **REIKI** cleanses the body of toxins.
- **REIKI** delivers according to the needs of the recipient.
- **REIKI** is effective on animals, plants and other various things.
- **REIKI** is an extremely pleasant method of healing.
- **REIKI** balances the energies of body.
- **REIKI** loosens up blocked energy and helps to attain a state of total relaxation.

Reiki can never do damage in any way, since it only flows in the quantities required by the recipient.

The effect of Reiki on the practitioner? What does he feel, what does he experience when he is treating someone with it? It has already been mentioned that the practitioners are only a channel for Reiki. They are not the source of this energy; rather they place us at its disposal as a kind of catalyst. No special kind of power or ability is necessary and no great effort is required. On the contrary, while they direct the flow of Reiki to a patient's body, they are being charged with it simultaneously.

The practitioner frequently experiences a sense of flowing in their hands. Some often have the feeling of sparks flying away from their hands, as if flashes of energy were jumping over to the patient. This is always a pleasant and harmonious experience for them. The experience the practitioner has above all is a deep feeling of inner union with the patient. One often intuitively senses a patient's deficiencies or disorders while he is treating him. Afterwards he feels happy and balanced physically and spiritually.

The treatment with Reiki can result in the appearance of a slight or more vehement detoxication symptom on the physical level. These symptoms are to be regarded as a biologically sensible means of self-regulation. They generally take on the form of increase evacuation of the bowels and urine, and increase mucus secretion in the upper respiratory tract, while burning tears in eyes may also occur. Sometimes ears and skin expel an increased amount of waste products. A temporary fever or a temporary return of an earlier illness are also possible. These occurrences are to be considered as a valuable means of recovering physical health and not as a return of illness representing as they do in absolutely natural cleansing mechanism. These reactions only last a short time, and the patient will generally feel all the better for them. It should be noted that after a long period of fasting, similar kind of symptoms appear.

It may look odd to some people that Reiki therapy may cause previous illnesses to reappear and run a shortened course with Reiki treatment, but the illnesses previously suffered are experienced briefly again in reverse order, signifying a genuine and natural healing a phenomenon that may occur as a result of Reiki treatment.

First of all, unresolved experiences and problems should be brought back to consciousness where they can be resolved and laid to one side as being over. In this manner, tensions, which are often rooted in the past and are the cause of blockages in the present, can be neutralized with the help of Reiki.

If one treats with Reiki to a great extent, similar reactions to the ones described above may happen to him, too. This is because when you treat someone with Reiki, it will be flowing through your hands and yourself, unfolding its healing power within you at the same time as the patient. Thus, by passing Reiki on to others, you yourself will be cleansed more and more and made whole and healthy. You will notice that trust will slowly begin to develop within you, trust in a wisdom and power that will stick to you the whole life. The Reiki will lead you to insight and knowledge, to a conscious sense of unity with the whole of universe and above all, it will fill you with love and joy.

# HISTORY OF REIKI

During mid-1800s Dr. Mikao Usui was the dean of a small Christian University in Kyoto, Japan. This was an exciting period in Japan's history and many changes were taking place throughout society. The Japanese had recently reopened their shores to the foreigners, and were quickly adopting all of the new technology for the industrial development. Dr. Usui had adopted Christianity whole heartedly, becoming a minister and then finally Dean of a Christian seminary.

One day, during a discussion with some of students, Usui was asked if he believed literally in the Bible. When he replied that he did, his students reminded him of the instant healings of Christ. The students mentioned that in the Bible, Christ states, "You will do as I have done, and even greater things. if this is so," they stated, "Why aren't there many healers in the world today performing the same acts as Christ? In addition, he tells the apostles to heal the sick and raise the dead. If this is true," the students said, "please teach us the methods." Usui was taken aback. In traditional Japanese style, he was bound by his honor as Dean, to be able to answer their questions. On that day Usui resigned with determination to find the answers to this great mystery. As most of his teachers had been American missionaries, and America was predominantly a Christian country, he decided to begin his study at the University of Chicago in the theological seminary. After a long period of study, in which he did not find his answers, Usui made up his mind to continue his research somewhere else.

Dr. Usui realized that Lord Buddha was also known to have performed incredible feats, so he decided to return to Japan, and see if he could indeed find some new or old information about more of the instantaneous types of physical healings,

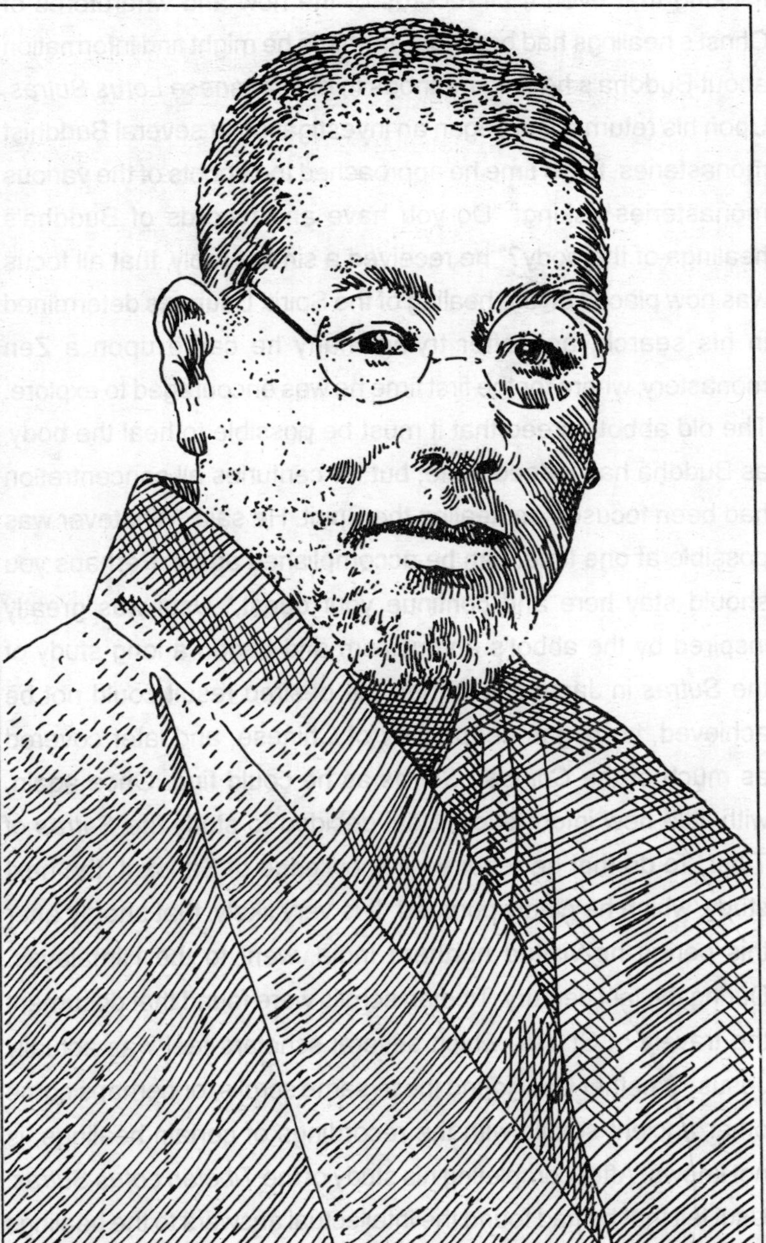

Dr. Mikao Usui

thinking that even if all records of the how and wherefores of Christ's healings had been lost, perhaps he might find information about Buddha's healing methods in the *Japanese Lotus Sutras*. Upon his return, Usui began an investigation of several Buddhist monasteries. Each time he approached the abbots of the various monasteries asking: "Do you have any records of Buddha's healings of the body?" he received a similar reply, that all focus was now placed on the healing of the Spirit. Usui was determined in his search, and after trying many he came upon a Zen monastery, where for the first time he was encouraged to explore. The old abbot agreed that it must be possible to heal the body, as Buddha had indeed done, but for centuries all concentration had been focused on healing the Spirit. He said "Whatever was possible at one time, can be accomplished again. Perhaps you should stay here and continue your quest," Usui was greatly inspired by the abbot's enthusiasm and began a long study of the *Sutras* in Japanese. When the desired result could not be achieved, he began deep study of Chinese, and later covered as much of the *Chinese Sutras* as he could find. Once again, with little new information, Usui decided to study the *Sutras of Tibet.* To do that he required a knowledge of Sanskrit, the next study, which he gladly pursued. It is very likely, that shortly after this period he visited northern India, went to the Himalayas. During the last century, Tibetan scrolls were found that document the travels of St. Isa, which several scholars feel was actually Jesus. Whether Usui found these same scrolls, or perhaps some other ancient scrolls with the recordings of certain healings, is not known. After completing his study of the *Tibetan Lotus Sutras,* Usui felt that he had found the intellectual answers to the healings of Christ. What he needed now was the empowerment.

After being sure that he had found the key to the mystery, Usui went back to the abbot to ask for advice on how to receive the actual empowerment. They both began to meditate, and together came to the conclusion that Dr. Usui should proceed to a sacred mountain about 17 miles from Kyoto, Mount Kuri Yama, and go through a 21-day fast and meditation.

Soon after that, Usui began his journey in the direction of mountain top. He came to a particular spot facing east, and gathered 21 stones which would be his calendar. After 20 days of fasting he arrived at the predawn of the 21st day. It was quite dark when he felt around for his last stone. Nothing out of the ordinary had happened up to this point. He prayed for the answer to come. In the sky he saw a flicker of light. It began to move very rapidly towards him. As it came closer it also got larger, Usui was frightened. He felt like getting up and running away. Finally, he realized this must be some sort of sign. He had sought so long and hard all of those years—he just couldn't give up. He gathered his courage for whatever might come, and momentarily the light struck him in the centre of his forehead. Usui thought he had died. Millions of rainbow coloured bubbles appeared before his eyes. Soon they turned into white glowing bubbles, each one containing a three-dimensional Sanskrit character in gold. They would appear one by one, just slowly enough for him to register each character. Finally, when it was over, Usui was filled with gratitude. As he had been in a trance-like state, he was surprised when he awakened and it was broad daylight. In his excitement to share his experience with his friend abbot, Usui began to run down the mountain. He was amazed at how strong and rejuvenated he felt, considering the long fasting period he had gone through. This was the first miracle of the morning. Suddenly, he tripped and stubbed his toe. He instinctively reached down and grabbed it, he was amazed to see that in few minutes, the bleeding stopped and it was completely healed—that was the second miracle of the morning. As he continued down the mountain, he came to a typical roadside stand, and ordered a heavy breakfast. As anyone knows, who is acquainted with fasting procedures, it is quite dangerous to break a long fast with a large meal. The proprietor could see by Usui's monk's garb, and unkempt beard, that he had been fasting and meditating, and suggested some special soup. Usui declined and ordered the full breakfast. The third 'miracle' of the morning occurred when he finished it without any digestive complication.

The old man's granddaughter who served food to Usui was in dire pain. She had a severe toothache and her jaw had been swollen for days. Her grandfather was extremely poor so he could not take her to a dentist in Kyoto, so when Usui offered to try and help, she gladly accepted. After he put his hands on the sides of her face, the pain and swelling began to disappear immediately.

Soon Dr. Usui was on his way to the monastery. He found the abbot in great pain due to arthritis. While Usui shared his experiences with the monk he laid his hands on the arthritic areas, and very quickly, the pain disappeared. The old abbot was truly amazed. Usui sought his advice as to what he should do with this new found ability. And finally after some discussion, he decided to go and work in the Beggars Quarter of Kyoto. He hoped to heal the beggars so that they could have new identity and secure a place in the society.

When Usui settled in the beggar quarter, he set about immediately, healing young and old alike. The results were remarkable and many were completely healed. After about seven years of this work, Usui noticed some familiar faces. One young man, who looked quite familiar, drew his attention. "Do I know you?" Usui asked.

"Why certainly!" the beggar replied, "I'm one of the first beggar you healed, I had a new identity, I found a job, and even got married. I just couldn't stand the responsibility. It's much easier to be a beggar."

Dr. Usui soon came across many similar cases. He wept in despair. Where had he gone wrong? It finally dawned on him that he had failed to teach them responsibility, and above all, the gratitude. He then realized that the healing of the spirit was as important as the healing of the body. He saw that by giving away Reiki he made beggars of people. He said "I cut off all beggars.Never again will Reiki be given away. Always the flow will have to be completed, Always there will have to be an exchange, with Reiki. And now I know how to heal the body and the spirit..."

At this time, Dr. Usui formulated the five principles of Reiki. He left the beggars quarter and began to teach Reiki throughout Japan. It was also at this time that the purpose of the symbols he had experienced in this vision became clear. He would use them to attune people so that they could take responsibility for their own well-being. By helping them amplify their energy, they could take a bigger step towards their own mastership. Usui began to train other teachers, young men who would join him in his travels and so started a tradition of apprenticeship in Reiki. On his travels he acquired 18 disciples. Dr. Usui had two children but they did not want to dedicate their lives to Reiki. Shortly before his transition, around the turn of the century, Usui chose one of his most devoted disciple. Dr. Chujiro Hayashi, a retired Naval officer to carry on the traditions of Reiki. Dr. Hayashi founded the first Reiki clinic in Tokyo which flourished for many years.

Hawayo Takata, a young Japanese-American woman from Hawaii appeared in Hayashi's clinic in 1935. She was very ill with a variety of organic disorders, and also lacking energy due to depression over the death of her husband a few years earlier. Having been on the verge of surgery while visiting her parents

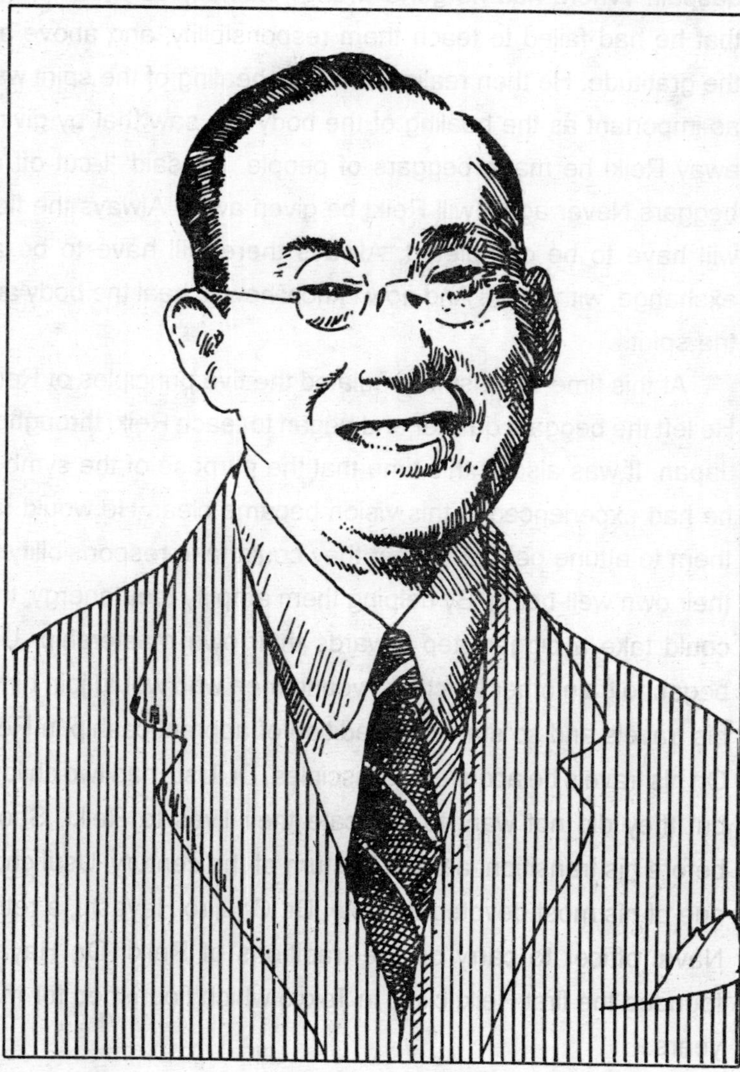

Dr. Chujiro Hayashi

who had returned to Japan, she heard a voice tell her the operation was not necessary. She thought that she was going crazy hearing voices when nobody was around when, for the third time she heard the voice, she asked that what should she do, she was told to 'ask the doctor'. After conferring to the doctor her reservations about the upcoming surgery, he recommended that she try the Reiki clinic, and it was there that she began to receive treatment, and within 8 months she was completely healed. Takata was quite impressed with Reiki and decided to learn it herself. Reiki had been a man's domain, and that was prohibited for women, particularly women belonging to the working class. Takata was a typical determined woman and did not give up easily. Her persistence ultimately paid off, and she was finally instructed in first degree techniques. Later Takata returned to Hawaii and began her practice. In 1938, Dr. Hayashi and his daughter came to visit her. Soon after, Takata was initiated as a Master and the Hayashis returned to Japan. In order to reach this level Takata had to sell her house for $10,000 to pay the fee, which Dr. Hayashi had set for Reiki Mastership.

In 1941, Dr. Hayshi saw that a war was inevitable with the U.S. and began to make preparations. Mrs. Takata sensed his concern and decided to return to Japan. Dr. Hayashi immediately warned her of the coming trouble. He already knew what the result of the war would be. He knew that Japan would be destroyed and that many would die. He warned Mrs. Takata of the preparations she would need to make in order to protect Reiki. Not wanting to be drafted to participate in the violence of the coming war, Dr. Hayashi decided to make his transition. One day in full ceremonial dress, and amidst friends, Hayashi consciously left his body. Takata pursued the teaching of Reiki in post-war America during the McCarthy era. This way Hawaii

Takata was chosen to hold in trust the sacred knowledge of Reiki after Dr. Hayashi.

In the 1970's Mrs. Takata began to train other Masters in USA and at the time of her death in December of 1980, 22 had been trained. Today there are over 300 Reiki Masters teaching around the world. Takata's granddaughter Phyllis Lei Furumoto is the current head of the Reiki lineage.

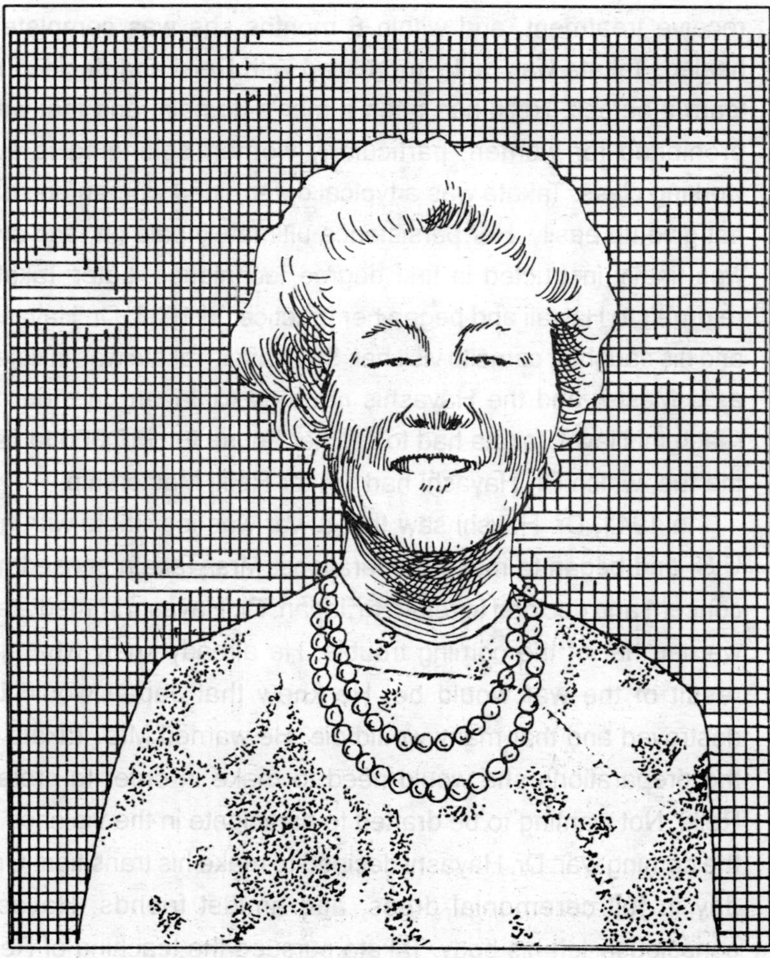

Madame Hawayo Takata

# LINEAGE OF REIKI MASTERS

Dr. Mikao Usui rediscovered Reiki in mid 1800's. Before his transition he trained Dr. Chujiro Hayashi.

Before his transition Dr. Hayashi trained and initiated Madame Hawayo Takata who initiated 22 Masters before her transition in 1980.

The Masters are:

1. George Araki
2. Dorothy Baba (transcended)
3. Ursula Baylow
4. Rick Bockner
5. Barbara Brown
6. Fran Brown
7. Patricia Ewing
8. Phyllis Lei Furomoto
9. Beth Grey
10. John Grey
11. Iris Ishikura (transcended)
12. Harry Kuboi
13. Ethel Lombardi
14. Barbara McCullough
15. Mary McFadyen
16. Paul Mitchell
17. Bethel Phaigh (transcended)
18. Barbara Weber Ray
19. Shinobu Saito
20. Virginia Samdahl (transcended)
21. Wanja Twan
22. Sister of Madame Takata

Only through direct connection to these 22 Masters is there true Reiki. The true Masters will never ever make 'Masters' of anyone who asks and pays their fee, so Reiki is worth carefully searching out the lineage of the person whom you consider as Master.

Just for today
I will give thanks
For my many blessings

Just for today
I will not worry

Just for today
I will not be angry

Just for today
I will do my work honestly

Just for today
I will be kind to my neighbour
and every living thing

Dr. Mikao Usui

# THE PRINCIPLES OF REIKI

The five principles of Reiki were developed by Dr. Usui shortly after he decided to leave the Beggars Quarter of Kyoto. He left Beggar City because he realized that Reiki fit differently into the world than he had first thought. It was at this time that he became aware of the some important aspects of human nature.

Dr. Usui had realized he had been treating only the physical disorders and had not been concerned with the spiritual, the exact opposite of his teaching experiences at the University. He had not taught the beggars gratitude. By giving away the Reiki, Dr. Usui had played into the mentality of the beggars, wanting something for nothing. They had not committed themselves to wanting the healing; they had not asked for it nor had they indicated its value to them by some exchange of energy. To live in gratitude is to live in abundance.

The casual factor must be sought in each individual. We cannot assume that what we want for another person, no matter how well-intentioned, is what is truly right for them, we might want a person to be cured so he does not experience pain or die. The truth is that despite our best intentions, we do not know what that person's soul path is meant to be. It is possible that his soul's choice is to die, using the illness to facilitate the process. Perhaps the pain, physical or emotional, is making the person learn a lesson. In addition, he may be getting some type of benefit such as attention from a loved one or financial support because of the illness and may not be ready to let it go. With Reiki, the requirement is that a person desire a healing and pay for it in an appropriate manner like fee or gratitude.

The channel through which affluence and harmony normally flow are either undeveloped or paralized, hence, the Reiki must be used in order to give to those channels their natural function. Our lessons in life come in many forms, and as with Dr. Usui, often our clarity only comes in hindsight. We sometimes handle thing as per our own thinking words, and actions, and usually we do it unknowingly, just as Dr. Usui did. Both Usui and the beggars learned much as a result of his seven years in beggar

City. On the surface, this experience would appear to some to be a failure, but we learn our lessons in numerous ways. Only through hindsight people can see the error of their ways.

The bad experiences inspired Dr. Usui to develop a set of principles which still hold true today. These principles are wonderful tools to assist in the growth process. The original Five Principles of Reiki as formulated by Dr. Usui are :

- Just for today I will give thanks for my many blessings
- Just for today I will not worry
- Just for today I will not be angry
- Just for today I will do my work honestly
- Just for today I will be kind to my neighbour and every living thing

## Just for today I will give thanks for my many blessings

So try to feel gratitude for everything in your life, the challenges as well as the joys, can transform your life. It has assisted many in changing their negative attitudes into positive ones. Reiki is one of the blessings of this lifetime that we can truly give thanks for on a daily basis. To truly live in a state of gratitude you must consciously look for the opportunity to thank someone or something. Reiki will assist in opening your consciousness so you can be aware of all that is around you just ready and waiting to be seen and appreciated. But for that a bit of discipline is needed to change old pattern and create a prosperous flow of Universal Life Force Energy.

## Just for today I will not worry

Worrying means overlooking that there is always a divine purpose for everything.

When you look at the positive side you will find that situations are not necessarily what they had appeared to be before. When one learns to take a positive attitude there will be less and less of the negative for him to see. Negative state of mind indicates a lack of faith in God who looks after us. Negativity and worry don't help anything they just hinder the outcome, and make us desperate in the meantime. Learn to do your best, leave the results for God, or the Power in which you have faith and you will find your approach more positive in the times to come.

## Just for today I will not be angry

Anger is totally an unnecessary emotion. To say we will not be angry is difficult, for there are some happenings and things in life that anger us. However, how we handle that anger is what is important. Anger is really a veil like emotion, usually covering up feelings of frustration, resentment or hurt. A major step forward in many people's growth path is learning to develop skills to uncover and deal with the emotions that are hidden behind this veil, and take action for change if that is required. When they can deal appropriately with the anger, their lives become much happier and easy.

## Just for today I will do my work honestly

To be honest with oneself is to face the truth in all things. Working honestly, whether for yourself or another, is crucial for good self esteem. One can sometimes fool other people with dishonesty, but one cannot fool himself. You are the one who must look at yourself in the mirror every night. Doing your work honestly, and in a larger sense living your life honestly, knowing that your ethics are clean whether anyone else appreciates it or not, brings you peace of mind, you can find no other way. To live ethically may be difficult but the serenity that results transforms people.

## Just for today I will be kind to my neighbour and every living thing

Kindness and love are insignificant without each other. Since we create our own worlds, hence, by being kind and loving everyone and everything, you will create a loving atmosphere for yourself to live in as well. We are all a collective energy from the same source, so we must get rid of self-centred tendency and learn to show respect for all life form to help heal the whole world.

# IS IT NECESSARY TO HAVE COMPLETE FAITH IN REIKI?

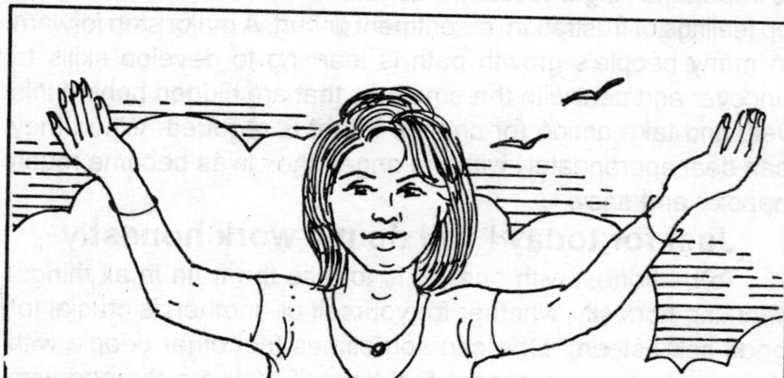

It is a very well-known fact if you believe in something it will help. Some people say that all these methods work when you have complete faith in them.

It means all people need to do to get healthy believe in anything, whether doctor, well wisher, medicine or religion. Why don't they do it then? Could it be that they don't believe in what they believe? Or they say it for argument sake. But what about the case when someone is unconscious and only conscious belief in something will cure him? What about infants and small children? How can animals and plants be treated with success if this is true? What should the practitioner do, if a patient tells him that he doesn't believe in his method or treatment?

It has been proved numerous times that Reiki will help in all these cases. *The American International Reiki Association* was founded a research institute where the steadily increasing amount of evidence proving the effectiveness of Reiki can be documented. Of course, it has not yet been possible to find satisfactory scientific explanations for all the miracles occurring due to Reiki, nor for its successes and apparent failures, but there are many things both in our lives and in the life of the universe that have not yet been scientifically explained and explored. For example, we do not know why the taste of mango is so delicious or why our galaxy functions without error. In spite of this, the mango delights us and we are nourished daily by the light of the sun and enjoy the sparkle of the stars. The fact that we are benefited by these things is enough for us so we continue to appreciate them in the future. The experience of Reiki alone will be sufficient to prove its worth, but science and belief also have their role to play. Science, for example, can confirm the effects that Reiki causes while believing in it can open us up to receive it better. Of course, Reiki will function without any preconceptions, but the presence of them won't harm or change anything.

Though it is also a fact that everything we do with inner happiness, conviction optimism and dedication will bring about success and fulfilment, no matter what the area of life is. This fact plays an inestimable role in all kinds of therapy too. If we are against a form of treatment whether due to our outer lifestyle or inner attitude, we will harm ourselves above all. We can even impede the natural flow of healing by having a negative outlook or attitude, it may cause some delay in healing.

Our bodies immediately react to our thoughts has been proved by means of simple kinesiological tests, which prove that as soon as we think negatively (or find ourselves in a negative situation), the organism reacts with weakness or reduced vitality. But the positive thoughts or situations increase strength and vitality. The influence of our spirit affects all aspects of our existence. With our fears and wishes, thoughts and feelings, words and deeds, both conscious and unconscious, we daily forge our lives.

Suppose if we produce a certain kind of thought only rarely or in a superficial manner, the elemental generated will not be very substantial and will immediately disappear. If we think of something very often or very intensely however, the corresponding elemental will become larger and stronger in accordance and will manage to stick for a long time.

This point should be noted that elemental possesses a certain *freedom of action*. It can take up contact with similar impulses coming from the surroundings in order to fulfil a *mother-thought,* such as *I feel great today.* In order to nourish itself and keep alive, the elemental will automatically do everything in its power to have this thought repeated and confirmed. This theory provides a plausible explanation for the great results achieved by various methods of positive thinking and approach.

The same is also applicable in the case of negative thoughts. We all know how difficult it is to give up a bad habit or stop repeating a certain thought or thinking about things in a certain way. The moment we try to do this by letting unwanted thoughts pass by unnoticed, the "elemental" in question tries to push us back to the desired way of thinking. But if it fails to do so it gets insubstantial gradually and soon vanishes altogether.

A particular segment or group of people may build up a thought of their own. The effect of such a collective thought can be quite overwhelming. The more people involved in it, the greater will be its effect. For example, what would happen if some agency raises false alarm about an influenza epidemic, with details of the symptoms. How many people would immediately feel unwell and get it?

But if the same people are told instead that, unusual weather conditions would increase their vitality and immunity to disease in the coming days. Would they get unwell?

The effect of collective thought can be increased further when the thought in question is taken up on a very peak level of consciousness. Just as the finer the form of matter, the more energy will be present there, so the closer we are to a state of inner unity with all creation, the more effective our thoughts will be.

At this stage, new laws come into force, laws which exceed by far the influence of the elementals. A thought of love expressed on this finest level of consciousness, where *Divinity* which is to be found in all beings, will be able to come into contact with the innermost sphere of life itself without needing the agency of an elemental. Hence, every thought made on this level will automatically be positive in every way.

The knowledge of cause and effect is practical reality for many people. For others, it is still very unusual, but the fact that a point of view is habitual, does not mean to say that it is the truth. If you wish to undergo Reiki treatment without being absolutely convinced of the effectiveness of the method, then take up a neutral attitude. You should have sufficient patience to wait and see what happens. Even if you do build up a negative thought elemental, it won't affect the ability of Reiki to heal you, but of course an open or positive attitude will open you to receive Reiki in a shorter time.

Reiki does not require great effort, talent or ability, it is a method of healing which is absolutely natural and it is this natural flow of life which leads us on to greater perfection, harmony and happiness.

In order to see the positive side of things, however, you will have to open yourself up first for Reiki; you will be surprised by its miraculous results.

# THE DIFFERENCE BETWEEN REIKI AND OTHER HEALING METHODS

The main highlight of Reiki is its simplicity. Where other forms of therapy may demand months and years of training for the healer, Reiki can be taught in a weekend. The real difference is in the attunement process which puts Reiki in the category of energy work and in a class of its own.

After going through the attunement process, most doctors, nurses, massage therapists, and people well-acquainted with the touch and feel of the human body, notice immediate increases in the amount of energy or the feeling of heat emanating from their hands when doing treatment. Thus people with prior experience of the body usually receive immediate feedback of the change which occurs as a result of the attunements, and the sensations which sometimes occur during the actual attunements. Others with less experience or sensitivity need time and practice doing treatments to learn to detect the changes immediately and act according to the need. Many people are able to do that, it is simply that those with too many preconceived notions need to learn how to listen to the body, because a successful treatment requires a listening process. The extensive amount of experiential time Reiki Masters allot to their students for practicing treatments, provides enough chance for feedback and verification that there are indeed different sensations being experienced by the "healer", if not as strongly initially by the practitioner.

Generally when a massage therapist is working on a client, and especially during deep tissue release work, it is necessary to keep the knees unlocked or slightly bent. This is because the therapist acts as a grounding rod to the client.

Suppose a healer is helping you release a large knot in your neck or shoulder, as he guides your breathing and you consciously release the lactic acid from the muscle, as long as his hands are on the knot, the negative energy being released runs into his hand, down his arm, and out of his feet into the ground. If ever he keeps his knees stiff or locked during this process, your energy runs down his arm and body, does an abrupt U-turn at his knees, and returns to the exact spot in his body which is being released in yours.

It would sound peculiar when you are first learning about the movement of energy in the body, but it only takes a few unconscious moments to learn the truth of this process. It was quite a surprise to find that with Reiki this is not a problem or concern, because Reiki is drawn by the healer through the open channel of the practitioner. The practitioner never absorbs energy from the healer, as the energy is always "outward bound" with the exception of what may be deposited and stored on the solar plexus. The healee, on the other hand, draws Reiki through a clear channel and thus does not absorb any of the personal energy of the practitioner/healer, this point should be understood clearly.

Reiki is a unique art of healing. In other forms of energy work such as magnetic or mental healing, the practitioner must concentrate hard on sending energy with no distraction from the client. In Reiki, once the initial intention to treat has been completed and the hands have been placed on the body, the energy will then be drawn of its own accord with no further intense focus from the practitioner needed. Thus, if a client wants to talk about something, the healer can hold a conversation and continue to treat simultaneously.

Some Masters always discourage their students from initiating any talk, because most of the times the client tends to process at a level beyond words, and talking would be a great interference in the process. This brings up an important aspect from a therapeutic standpoint.

Many times, the same people return time and again with a different form of one basic problem. The more they would dwell on it verbally, the more it became "ingrained in the brain". Instead of releasing the problem, it may intensify the problem. Of course, a good psychologist or counsellor is trained to help turn negative ideas into positive ones, and help the person release the pattern. With Reiki, much of the verbal release is unnecessary. During and shortly after a treatment, and especially throughout the

21-day cleansing period, after receiving either of the three degrees, people have a tendency to feel emotions bubbling to the surface. That makes people more talkative.

One should acknowledge these emotions which sometimes appear unexpectedly, and feel gratitude towards them (the emotions) for showing themselves and to let them go. By not suppressing them, but acknowledging them in a very conscious way, they seem to vanish pretty soon.

The people should know the importance of letting emotions go. For example, a person who after a long period of depression, finally moves to a stage where anger begins to be released. As anger is a higher vibratory energy than depression, the person may develop a tendency to enjoy the expression of anger without then moving on to a higher level of expression. Anger can be very seductive, because all of the drama involved really stimulates the ego to a high pitch. Anger is a result of feeling out of control. It is a result of failing to realize and take responsibility for all that we have created in our lives. It is so important to understand that you would pluck what you would sow.

Like other therapies Reiki seeks to help each individual find balance and harmony in the body, mind and spirit. Reiki is truly a gift to you, the power to co-create is your birthright. With that power comes the privilege of greater responsibility, and one must perform his duty with sincerity and modesty.

# THE EFFECTS OF REIKI TREATMENT

Reiki amplifies and balances *Energy,* increases *Awareness* and *Creativity,* helps release *Emotions,* and *Stress* works on casual level of *Disease* and *Heals.*

The results of every Reiki treatment are determined by the needs of the person being treated. The style of each Reiki healer may be different, but the primary focus of every healer will be on troublesome area of the body and the endocrine system.

Mrs. Hawayo Takata taught a basic treatment pattern which covered all of these very important glandular systems, which in turn control the hormones of the body. To orthodox medicine, these glands are stimulated by neuro transmitters. The body communicates with the nervous system through the brain, which then stimulates the glands to release hormones that are needed for homeostasis. On the etheric level, each of the seven main chakras, or energy centres, corresponds to one of the endocrine glands (shown in the following figure).

Thus, the endocrine system acts as a transducer of energy to the etheric energy centres, or chakras, and likewise the chakras act as devices that convert energy back to the physical system through the endocrine glands. All levels are in some way interconnected with each other.

The flaws which have roots in structural defects are generally caused by chemical imbalance, they demand repair procedure for adjustment of the chemical environment (via drugs in man, or fertilizers in the case of agriculture). The dilemma that occurs is that both the organism (body or plant) and its threatening invaders adapt to the new chemical complex, in turn becoming less sensitive to it, so that an increased amount of potency is required everytime. The unnatural chemical content of the organism thus increases and begins to influence other levels of functioning, not only the one being corrected, but other levels also, its results can be disastrous.

The deadly effect of this kind of procedure can be seen in agriculture, where many people die from high levels of toxic poisoning. In medicine, this type of procedure had resulted in many people suffering from diseases caused by the doctors. Now most of the physicians are aware of this deadly problem and are adopting more preventative methods to avoid

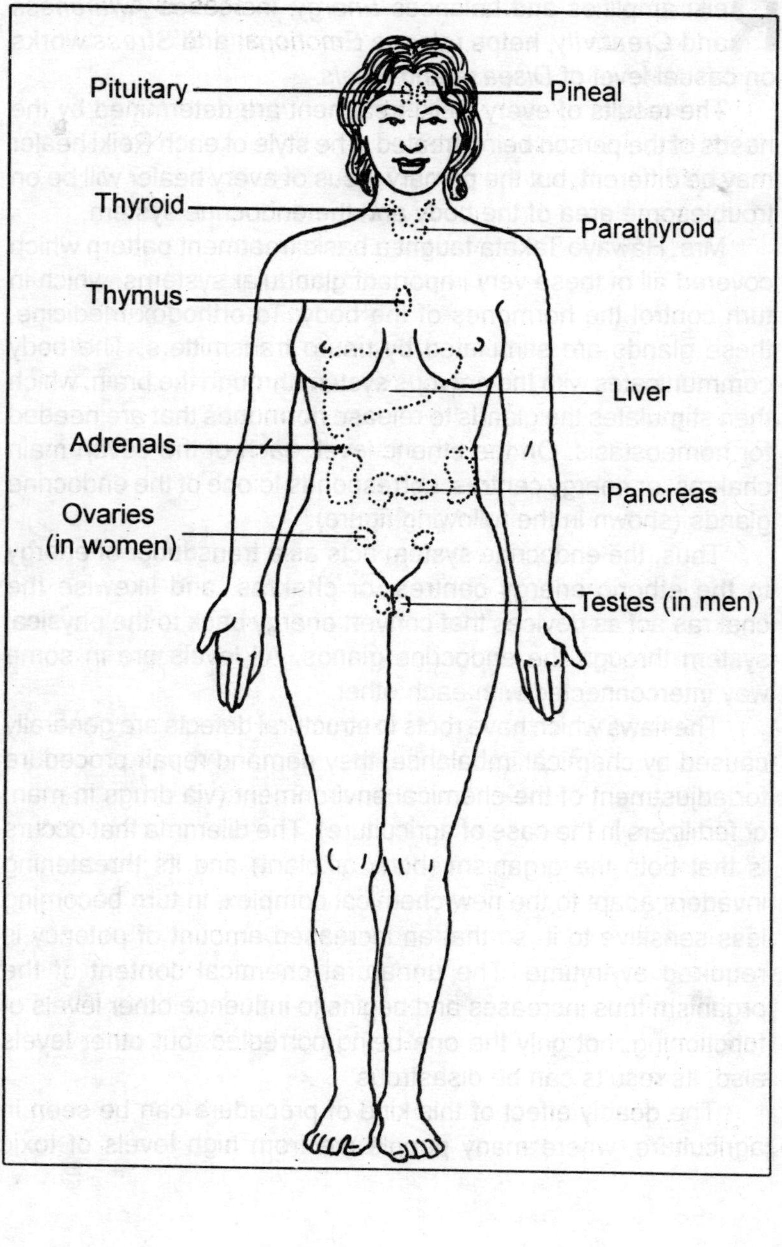

complications caused by increased quantity of medicine or over exposure to X-rays, etc.

The Reiki practitioners are always able to recognize the harmony of the etheric and physical bodies through the connection of the chakras and endocrine system. Besides that, the 'Second Degree Reiki' gives the practitioner additional knowledge to help deal with the mental level of disease, where the causal factor is found. It is quite obvious to Reiki practitioners that the causal level of disease rests with the mind.

The Reiki energy naturally works on the physical, mental and etheric levels. Reiki helps each individual release energy blocks and the connected emotions, which in turn helps the release of the causal level of disease. If the root cause would be gone, then there would not be any danger of serious complication.

# THE ATTUNEMENTS

Some day a person who had Reiki may feel the desire to not only receive Reiki but pass it on to others as well. Maybe you have had Reiki treatment and now want to use it on yourself. You must be curious to know about the requirement. Here is a brief description of basic requirements.

Attunements are the very core of the Usui method of natural healing. Reiki is the Japanese word for Universal Life Force Energy, something which we all have as our birthright. Anyone can lay hands on another person and transmit magnetic Life Force Energy. What makes Usui's system unique is the attunement process, which may be described as a series of initiations wherein a Reiki Master, using a very ancient *Tibetan technology,* transmits energy to the student in an amplified state. The energy acts in such a way that it creates an open channel for cosmic energy to flow in from the top of the student's head, through the upper energy centres and out through the hands, for use in future treatments. In addition, the vibratory rate of the body is amplified, triggering a 21-day cleansing period, which occurs as a result of negative patterns and blocks being sloughed off due to the quickening of a person's energy pattern.

Reiki is so easy to learn that children will learn it in two days. However, the desire to use Reiki for the benefit of yourself and others should be an honest one and not the result of a passing whim or fancy. Once you are quite clear on this, you will learn this unique art of healing within no time.

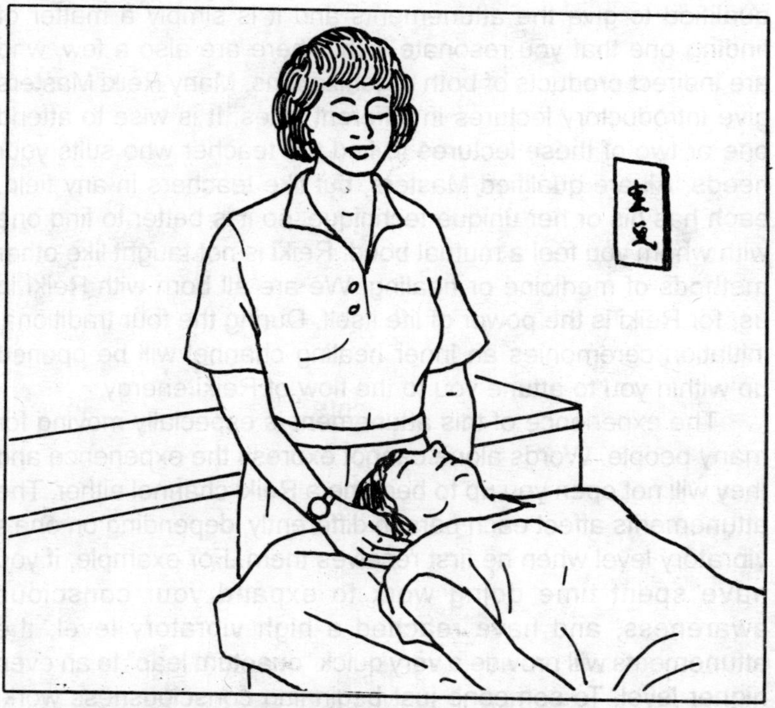

As per the original tradition of Reiki there are two Reiki degrees as well as a Master degree. This tradition was represented uniformly by both Reiki organizations until 1983. The First Degree will enable you to transfer Reiki to yourself and others by the laying on of your hands. This degree can be obtained in the weekend course. The First Degree course usually begins with some introductory explanations and then the first of four initiations or attunements.

The attunements are very precise and can only be transmitted by a Reiki Master who has been trained in Dr Usui's method. There are two main schools of Reiki. One is headed by Phyllis Lei Furumoto, who is Mrs. Takata's granddaughter, and is called the *Reiki Alliance*. Several of the original 22 Reiki Masters trained by Takata are members of this group. The other organization, called the American International Reiki Association (AIRA), is headed by Dr. Barbara Weber Ray, and for the past couple of years, has used the term "The Radiance technique" for describing Reiki. Reiki Master from either group are fully qualified to give the attunements and it is simply a matter of finding one that you resonate with. There are also a few, who are indirect products of both organizations. Many Reiki Masters give introductory lectures in different cities. It is wise to attend one or two of these lectures to find the teacher who suits your needs. All are qualified Masters, but like teachers in any field, each has his or her unique technique, so it is better to find one with whom you feel a mutual bond. Reiki is not taught like other methods of medicine or healing. We are all born with Reiki in us, for Reiki is the power of life itself. During the four traditional initiation ceremonies an inner healing channel will be opened up within you to attune you to the flow of Reiki energy.

The experience of this attunement is especially moving for many people. Words alone cannot express the experience and they will not open you up to become a Reiki channel either. The attunements affect each person differently, depending on one's vibratory level when he first receives them. For example, if you have spent time doing work to expand your conscious awareness, and have reached a high vibratory level, the attunements will provide a very quick "quantum leap" to an even higher level. To someone just beginning consciousness work, there is also a "quantum leap" but the expansion of energy will be relative to the level that you start out with. The wonderful thing about Reiki is that, even after the "Quantum leap" which is caused by the attunements, you can still continue to increase your vibratory level and healing capacity by treating yourself daily, treating others whenever possible and meditation.

The main aim of First Degree attunements is opening up the physical body so that it can then accept (channel) greater quantities of life force energy. The four attunements of First Degree raise the vibratory rate of the four energy centres of the upper part of the body, which are also known as *chakras.* The first initiation attunes both the heart and the thymus while also attuning the heart chakra on the etheric level. The second attunement affects the thyroid gland, and on an etheric level, helps to open up the throat chakra, which is the communication centre. The third initiation affects both the third eye, which corresponds to the pituitary gland. The centre of higher consciousness and intuition, and the hypothalamus, which affects the body's mood and temperature. The fourth initiation further opens the Crown Chakra, our connecting link with spiritual consciousness, and it's corresponding physical partner, the pineal gland. This final attunement completes the process by sealing the channel open, so that you can maintain the accelerated ability to channel the Reiki energy for the rest of your life. Thus it is essential to complete all four attunements to keep the Reiki channel open throughout your entire lifetime. Once you are attuned to the Reiki energy, you can never lose it. Even if you don't use it for a period of 30 years, the moment you decide to use it, it will be there to use as it was 30 years ago.

After the First Degree initiation, Reiki energy will start to flow through your hands. The Master may have told you to put your hands on yourself beforehand and watch what happens. When you do the same thing afterwards, you will notice a definite difference, for a fine form of energy will be flowing through your hands, pleasant, warm and healing.

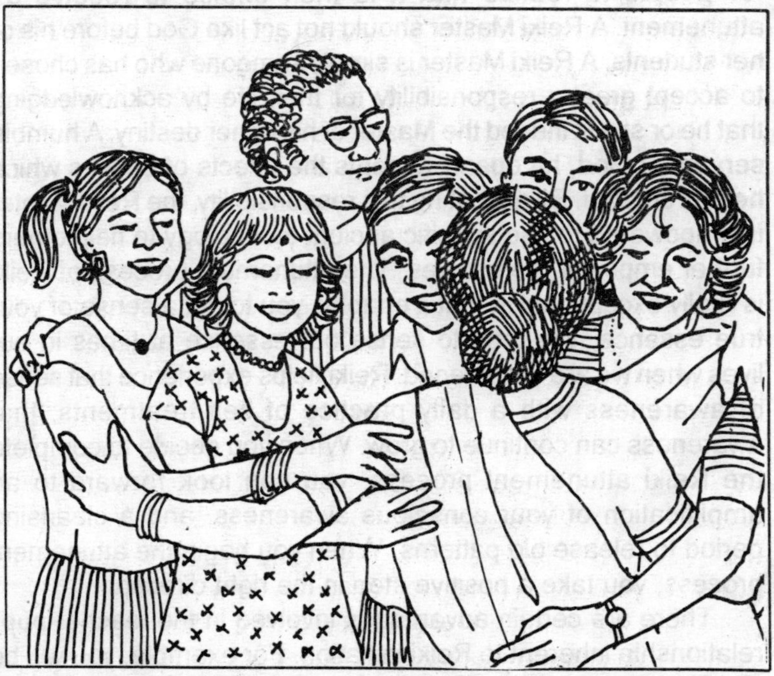

Before the seminar comes to an end, you will be handed out First Degree Certificates and everyone will probably embrace before the group finally breaks up.

Second Degree attunement process provides an amazing leap in vibratory level, at least four times greater than First Degree. The three symbols which are taught in Second Degree, to be used for sending absentee healings, also become activated at this point. Second Degree has great emphasis on adjusting the etheric body, rather than the physical body, which is the primary focus of First Degree. In addition the third eye or sixth chakra is greatly affected, which often heightens the intuitive abilities of the student. Soon after the Second Degree attunements, and especially during the 21-day cleanse process, people often feel a considerable amount of energy in their root chakras, because their survival and sexual centers become very stimulated.

Third Degree attunement is used to initiate a Master. This attunement again amplifies the vibratory level and activates the Master symbol so it may be used to help others empower themselves. This is an important point, because it is essential for people to realize that it is their choice to receive an attunement. A Reiki Master should not act like God before his or her students. A Reiki Master is simply someone who has chosen to accept greater responsibility for their life by acknowledging that he or she is indeed the Master of his or her destiny. A humble servant of God, he openly accepts the effects of causes which he has created. By accepting this responsibility, the Reiki Master is empowered to use specific ancient technology to help others further empower themselves. The attunement process of Reiki is really exceptional in that it enables you to get a sense of your true essence. We tend to sense our essence at times in our lives when we are enlightened. Reiki helps experience that sense of awareness with a daily practice of self-treatments, that awareness can continue to grow. When you decide to complete the Reiki attunement process, you can look forward to an amplification of your conscious awareness, and a cleansing period to release old patterns. When you begin the attunement process, you take a positive step in the right direction.

There are certain advantages involved in the teacher-pupil relationship inherent to Reiki initiation. For example, you will be able to ask the teacher for his advice if you are baffled at some function. Furthermore, your teacher would be part of a traditional line of Masters who have preserved the true knowledge of Reiki in its original form over a long period of time, thus it ensures both the purity and effectiveness of what you learn.

Reiki seminars are now held at regular intervals in many cities and exact details can be obtained from any of the Reiki Masters. Get further detailed information from the associations. That way you will know their differences and schedules, so that you may choose the suitable one.

Though their are various organisations, but the Reiki Alliance continues the traditional teaching of two degrees and a Master's degree, while since 1983 the A.I.R.A. (now T.R.T.A.I.) has made changes and modifications in the way of teaching, in the division and number of degrees and in the naming of Reiki and their organization. If you would like to be informed about the current situation, you may contact the organization directly. The addresses are given at the end of this book for your convenience.

# THE CLEANSE PROCESS AND TRANSFORMATION TOOLS

Some students are led to do cleansing and purification rites before taking Reiki, but it is not necessary, though if they do it there is no harm and it can be excellent for some students. After the attunement process in each of the three degrees, the student will undergo a 21-day cleanse process. Due to the raised vibratory rate of the physical and etheric bodies, old dense negative energy is forced to appear on surface, and is released. Everything is composed of energy, hence, everything has a vibration. In a similar fashion, negative blocks and emotional patterns, which are stored in our physical and etheric bodies, have a lower vibratory rate than the thought waves or stores of energy that we create when we are having positive thoughts. Thus, as we increase our vibratory rate, through steady persistence at whichever spiritual discipline we choose to study, we begin to notice how much easier it is to maintain a positive flow by simple methods.

After having a series of Reiki attunements, the sudden amplification of vibratory rate would set off an accelerated loosening of negative, dense energy within our systems, which cannot resonate with the finer vibrations created by the attunements. Since your vibration is adjusted so quickly, a reaction takes place which allows old stored-up emotions and memories to be released, as is appropriate for further growth. Although the change is sudden, it takes time for the adjustments to become effective. It takes approximately three-four days for the energy to move through each of the seven main chakras. Although the opening of the Reiki channel occurs between the heart center and the Crown Chakra, the centers in the lower part of the body are equally important and go through a corresponding adjustment in vibratory rate.

As a result of cleansing process some typical outward signs can be noticed in the life, like strange feelings, many kinds of dreams, emotional and physical changes such as detoxification, and attitude towards favourite food, which loses its importance in your life. These are just a few of the possible symptoms of the change which occurs at different levels of the physical and etheric bodies. Some reactions may seem unpleasant at first, as the negative energy is released, but by just facing each experience with use of willpower taking it in stride and not attaching a great deal of concern, each one will simply pass away and teach you something.

The students must keep a journal during this process to record the changes which occur. Besides that, note down details of your dream first thing in the morning. You will find that after a week of persisting with this suggestion, that your dream retention increases dramatically. Dreams are a wonderful tool to help us tune in with our subconscious. Although they may seem nonsensical or unclear at first, but gradually a pattern will begin to emerge. It is good also, at this time, to develop a habit of giving yourself Reiki treatments before you fall asleep at night, and first thing after you wake up in the morning after noting down your dream. If you continue to treat yourself after the initial cleanse process is completed, you will help the growth process to continue, and further refinement of your energy will take place. As you release old undesired feelings and concepts, you will begin to feel the attitude of gratitude flow naturally in your mind, which will in turn create a greater level of abundance with which you will live forever.

## POINTS TO REMEMBER

- All the positions given in the chapter Self-Treatment should be followed daily during cleanse process.
- Self-treatment positions no. 4, 6, 8, 9, 13 and 27 should be followed daily to remain in lush of health.

# TRANSFORMATION TOOLS

Reiki is doubtlessly the finest tool for transformation. There are many tools to be used with Reiki to accelerate the transformation and growth process.

## MEDITATION

Meditation is one of the most important tool for transformation. Meditation is like listening to the answers. These answers may come in many forms like overhearing someone else's conversation, dreams, a song, etc.

There are various ways of meditation, and you must choose the suitable one for yourself.

## PRAYER

The prayer is like talking to God or Supreme Power when you will start praying (if you were not doing it before) you will find that your meditation and prayer time become an important part in your daily routine.

Combination of prayer and meditation will change your life completely.

## PURIFICATION AND DETOXIFICATION

Purification and Detoxification are important to be in sound physical and mental conditions.

For detoxifying do not forget to drink water at regular intervals, so that the toxins can be flushed out of your system.

Deep breathing is another effective way for detoxification it would be much better if you find a yoga teacher and learn the correct technique from him.

To accelerate the removal process in case of water soluble toxins you may try Epsom Salt baths. Mix 2 kg. epsom salt in very hot water, as hot as you can tolerate. Spend 20 to 30 minutes in the tub, then take a shower, get into bed and sleep. You will definitely feel great next morning. This therapy will take care of symptoms of cold or flue also

## POSITIVE THOUGHTS

To change negative thought process into a positive one generally takes some time and needs some extra effort, but it can be done by reading right kind of books, listening to positive thought tapes and mixing with positive people.

Reiki is extremely helpful in releasing the negative to make room for the positive.

# THE FIRST DEGREE

You would be curious to know that why there are different degrees in Reiki. During Usui's time, students would travel with him, slowly becoming initiated in the various levels of energy until they too could become teachers. In modern times, the division of attunements into degrees has made it easier to get accustomed to the various stages of energy amplification. Before completing each successive step, it is good to give each student an adequate period of time to adjust to the higher vibratory level, and master the uses of the specific level. During the First Degree class, the student receives a permanent attunement to the Reiki energy, which occurs through four initiations. These initiations help to adjust the vibratory level of the recipient so that more energy can be channeled through the body. Due to this, adjustment also takes place on the etheric level which one can notice soon.

Though Reiki can produce miraculous results, but it is a very simple technique when it comes to application. There is no requirement of intellect in learning Reiki, thus, even children can learn it in the normal two-day class duration. First Degree is usually taught in three-four hour sessions. Initially the student is given the history and related background of Reiki, as well as the basic hand positions for self-treatment. The first two attunements are then given and each person begins to do a self-treatment. It is at this point that people discern the difference between before the attunement, and after the attunement, by the increase in either heat, tingling or pulsations, which begin to be felt in the hands. But remember the attunements give you Reiki.

In the second session you will learn about exercises for developing kinesthetic sensitivity, after which the positions are given for laying hands on another. The remaining time is then spent on group treatments. The students then begin to feel the differences in energy drawn by each individual. Each student also gets an opportunity to experience a treatment from the group of healers.

The third session starts with the final two attunements of the First Degree. Later there is discussion about the different feelings and experiences that the participants have with the attunements. At this point, students are asked to keep a 21 day journal, as it is good to take note of the changes that occur, so that one can refer to them later for a greater sense of verification whether the Reiki process does indeed facilitate cleansing and healing. The students should also begin a self-remembering exercise each evening before going to sleep.

Most of the people are not aware that in truth they are all in a type of hypnotic trance 24 hours a day. Hypnosis itself is only a tool to help concentrate the mind on one thing at a time. Though, most people experience the physical effect of loss of peripheral vision, while under hypnosis. They become truly one-sighted. During most of our normal waking hours, we are hypnotized by our conditioning. We experience a broader view in our normal lives than under induced hypnosis, but our concentration is on old patterns of behaviour.

Most of us, most of the time, are not really experiencing life, we are reacting to life by plugging into old patterns of response. We need to look at life as fresh and new each day. We need to learn again to experience life as it truly happens, without allowing preconceived notions or old patterns of response, which can often cause us to misinterpret the truth in many of life's situations.

It takes a great deal of conscious effort and discipline to break free of our old patterns. There must be a willingness to review one's actions each day, and see what could have been done better. What old habits need to be changed? Actually you will find that some patterns of behaviour, such as good manners, are quite positive. What we can add to these positive patterns, to make them even more effective, is our conscious awareness. In other words, when you say "Hello" to a stranger, don't just mumble it out of habit. Look the person in the eye and connect. You will feel so much more alive, and will help the other person to feel the same way. When you walk down a crowded area, consciously send love out to those around you — it will make a difference. When you make a conscious effort to "wake up", others around you will tend to pick it up by osmosis. The wave of gratitude will flow through you, and with practice staying consciously aware, will seem more effortless.

For rapid personal growth, it is beneficial to do a nightly self-evaluation. Review your day mentally and think back to how you reacted to each person and situation. What was appropriate and what could have been changed? What do you remember most clearly? You will find that the memories in life, which you recall so clearly, are from circumstances which occurred when you had a flash of conscious awareness. This exercise will help you to become aware of your behaviour. With practice, you will begin to see yourself, watch yourself and catch yourself before applying an old inappropriate approach in new circumstances.

There is another issue which is discussed in the First Degree class, that is helping people deal with a healing crisis. To begin with, whenever starting treatment on someone, it is recommended that there should be a commitment from the healee to receive a minimum of three treatments in succession, over a three-day period, if possible. There is often a gap of approximately three days for energy to be transmuted from the physical body to the etheric body, and vice versa. It is ideal to continue successive treatments during this period. As a result, if you are working on a person with an acute illness, they may experience more pain in the first two or three days of treatment, due to the acceleration of healing energy. The pain then seems to dissipate quickly on the third day. Hence, it is good to warn the patient that he might experience the illness more intensely at first, but that will be a temporary phase, and he will feel better after that.

If one is working on a person with a chronic illness, or one that has been active for a long time (such as asthma), you will find that Reiki usually brings immediate relief. When treatments are continued on chronic illnesses, the patient will usually feel steady improvement for quite some time. In this type of case, if there is to be healing crisis at all, it will usually occur several weeks after treatment. This is because the toxins, which caused the illness in the first palace, are slowly released until the point when they only have one final fortified place in the body. It seems that the last toxins or vestiges of a problem are the hardest to remove. Sometimes, when a person gets to this stage, he will experience the symptoms of the illness more intensely than ever before. It is at this time that healer must reassure the patient that the symptoms are a good sign of final release of the toxins. Additional treatments should be added at this time, to speed the release of toxins. It is better not to warn people with chronic illnesses about the symptoms of healing crisis, because you may project a response in them that might not otherwise occur. If it does occur however, you are forewarned and can reassure them that it is a very normal reaction, and help dissipate their fears. Again, in case of an acute illness, it is good to warn the patient that they may experience sensations that occur as a result of a rapid physical response to the illness, but that is quite a normal reaction.

If there is any serious acute crisis, a person should be referred to a qualified physician. Your treatments will then help to accelerate the healing as the healee draws only the energy needed to promote quick recovery. In the case of a chronic illness, the healee will most likely have already visited a physician. Your treatments will help to release toxins which have probably built up over a long period of time and needed to be expelled at the top priority.

The time period for getting rid of acute or chronic illnesses with Reiki is not definite. Each person is unique in the way that they react to treatments. Each person truly heals himself. Reiki channels act only as vessels through which healees draw the energy they need to create balance on all levels of their beings. It is not appropriate for us to place attachments on the results of our work, or to make any judgements, as each person accepts the amount of energy appropriate to his or her needs, and the results of the healing are not always directly visible. We must always keep in mind that there are often secondary benefits to having a disease, and a person may not be ready to be healed on the physical level due to disharmony between etheric and physical bodies. In the fourth session of the class, each student gives and receives a complete one hour Reiki treatment with a partner. Treating one person's whole body helps the student begin to discern between the differences in heat which are drawn in different areas of a body. Each person has different needs, and will draw different amounts of energy in different areas accordingly. The student then learns to give more attention to areas of the body which are drawing more energy. Finally, students again proceed with group treatments until each person has had a turn being treated. Then there is a final question and answer session. First Degree certificates are then awarded with the certificate you will have gained the ability to treat both yourself and others by the laying on your hands. You will also be able to increase the efficacy of medicine and strengthen the wholesomeness of food, cosmetics, etc., with the help of your Reiki energy as well as being able to transfer its healing power to animals and plants as well.

The students are also encouraged to continue meeting in groups to share treatment. During these first try-outs some participants may have some very moving experiences while others will simply feel relaxed and harmonious. Afterwards you will tell each other what you experienced and speak to the Master. During the course of the seminar you will notice how the facial expressions of the participants change, how they look younger and more relaxed. Every individual is special and brings their unique energy into the group. But keep it in your mind that 'ATTUNEMENTS' which work on electromagnetic field of the body align your Chakras and give you the REIKI.

Once obtaining the First Degree, a time of trying Reiki out will begin. You would be surely knowing someone you would like to treat.

# THE SECOND DEGREE

The Second Degree builds on the foundation laid in the First Degree. The Second Degree class provides the participant with the opportunity to attune to higher levels of the Reiki energy. The initiations of Second Degree also attune a person to the power keys or symbols, which are used at this level to perform absentee and a stronger form of mental/emotional healing. As Second Degree activates another level of energy (an amplification of vibratory level in both the physical and etheric bodies). The students will again go through 21-day cleanse period, similar to the one experienced in connection with First Degree, as their body and different energy centers adjust to an even finer level of vibration. Additional techniques for their personal growth can also be learnt at this stage.

The attunements in the First Degree concentrate on elevating the energy of the physical body, so that it may channel more intense healing energy, whereas Second Degree attunements work more directly on the etheric (bioplasmic) body and tend to stimulate development of the intuitive center which is located at the pituitary gland. Hermetic Science recognizes the pituitary gland to be the telepathic apparatus of the human body. It is known as the third eye. The pituitary gland is infinitely delicate and sensitive, and acts as a sending and receiving station for mental vibrations. After receiving Second Degree attunements, it seems that the normal spherical waves of thought which emanate from this center, and normally dissipate easily, are sharpened and become more easily focused in both their incoming and outgoing functions. Hence, gradually, it becomes easier for a Second Degree student to receive information on an intuitive level and that makes Reiki more simple to learn for him.

While the First Degree attunements align you, the Second Degree attunements empowers you. The development of intuition is vital, because it serves as the mouthpiece of our Higher Selves. By listening and reacting to the voice of his Higher Self one can find that he is on our proper life path and in a harmonius flow with those around him. Life then becomes rhythmatic and all of his activities become synchronized. The Higher Self truly knows everything, as it is not limited by time or space, and it does not need reason or logic to aid in its activities. Intuition knows because it simultaneously embraces cause and effect, the past, present and future. If one follows intuition, he will find that he ends up with positive results, even if it sometimes seems to argue with the conclusions of the intellect. In order to further develop intuition, we must learn to differentiate between the voice of desires placed in our minds by mass consciousness and those placed by our Higher Selves. One simple way to discriminate between the two is to notice the very different feelings that are evoked by inappropriate desires, and by those of the Higher Self. When the voice of intuition speaks to one, a sense of peace and harmony is evoked, even in a seemingly disharmonious situation, while inappropriate desires tend to bring on an unsettled feeling. Thus, it is better to listen to the voice of peace and wisdom, which brings a sense of harmony, than to heed the aggressive clamour of inappropriate desires, which only lead to ultimate dissatisfaction. The more one listens to his intuition, the more it develops. With practice, it becomes easier to follow the guidance of one's Higher Self, and increase one's confidence and wisdom. Second Degree gives a powerful boost to the development of this sixth sense. The Second Degree is a major tool in the transformational process for those who are on fast track of spiritualism.

Some of the sacred knowledge of Reiki is imparted to you at this level. In the Second Degree class, you are taught three keys which help to focus your mind so that it can send the Reiki energy beyond time and space. These keys unlock the Reiki power for those who have received the Second Degree initiations. There is nothing magical about the keys. They serve only as focus points for the practitioner's mind, to enable the Reiki energy to be channeled over long distances, and to amplify it for mental/emotional healing. The basis for the keys is found in age old universal laws that concern the transference of energy through the use of the mind. Because most thoughts are sent out like rays of light darting from a central point, they tend to lose much of their original force as they spred out — much like the waves created by throwing a pebble into still water. In contrast, to send a thought over a great distance, it must be concentrated, made one-pointed. The Reiki keys are the answer that Dr Usui found, which immediately enables a Second Degree practitioner to "send" the Reiki energy across time and space. To say that the energy is sent is, in a sense, a misnomer. Even in Second Degree the energy is drawn by the healee, not sent by the healer. With the keys, the pracitioner actually forms a "bridge" between himself and the healee, so that the energy can then be drawn when it is required.

The Second Degree class is usually taught on a weekend over three evenings. On the first evening, the keys and most of the intellectual information are passed on, in addition to the actual attunements. On the second evening, much of the time is spent learning to apply the keys and a special technique that promotes healing on the mental level. The third evening is focused primarily on absentee healing. A variety of possibilities for using the keys are discussed, and the student is encouraged to further explore these possibilities practically.

The Second Degree allows you to do special treatments on mental, emotional and addictive problems. The mental emotional healing technique helps to release the negative conditioning from past experiences. Very often, we react to certain circumstances in a negative way. When similar circumstances arise, instead of approaching them with an open mind, we usually react in a way which is called "pattern", even if such a reaction is inappropriate. Negative experiences themselves also tend to make us act in unconscious ways. Sometimes we find ourselves reacting to situations without any forethought. One of the Reiki keys, when used properly, helps to release these old patterned behaviour.

Reiki must be used to bring harmony and balance. Most of the time, physical illness is caused by the mind being out of synchronization with the spirit. There is much movement and growth which takes place as a result of taking the Second Degree Reiki class. The student should be prepared to experience change on several different levels. The changes which come, result in the empowerment of the student. With the empowerment comes greater responsibility, which is rewarded with greater healing power. Second Degree provides an opportunity to become consciously aware at a higher level. To take a Second

Degree class is to become aware of further dimensions of one's Higher Self. A greater sense of wholeness, peace and harmony results when the voice of intuition guides one.

You should always remember that the more Reiki you give, the stronger will be the energy flowing through you hands. Therefore, use Reiki as often as you can, to your own benefit and to that of others.

# THE THIRD DEGREE

The Master Level or Third Degree is final level of Reiki. Originally, Mastership was only for those dedicated to teaching Reiki. But today more and more people became interested in going beyond the Second Degree, although they know that they would probably never be chosen to become Masters. Hence many are allowed to have some of this advanced knowledge for their own personal growth and development.

At a Reiki Center a minimum of one year of working with the Second Degree energy is required before one can petition to be accepted for this advanced level of study. Master Teacher is the final level of Reiki Mastership. It is for those dedicated to teaching Reiki and to devoting their lives to Reiki. Masters are fully trained in the activations of First and Second Degree practitioners.

Minimum one year working with the Master Therapist is required before the initiating Master would consider a possible candidate for this level. At this level one is chosen, as has been practised in Oriental systems since ages.

# PRACTICAL WORK WITH REIKI

You cannot harm others and yourself with Reiki. A little Reiki is better than no Reiki. Here are some general rules and principles which should be observed when giving Reiki.

In the First Degree seminar you may learn various positions which are useful for giving treatment. There are about 10-20 basic positions alogether and a few additional ones for special cases. They are so logical and easy to carry out that they can be memorized by anyone in a couple of days. You will also be given a few sketches during most courses which will help refresh your memory, when necessary, while giving details of positions which have proved useful in the case of certain complaints and illnesses. And remember that there is no such thing as too much Reiki. The positions do not have to be carried out exactly as shown and it is not necessary to keep to the exact sequence either, although doing so will entail certain advantages. For example, you won't have to keep wondering which position comes next, or whether one has been forgotten, while you are treating a patient but will be free to concentrate on the patient and the way you are treating him, though Reiki can be effective even when the practitioner or the client is talking, laughing, crying, etc.

Let yourself be guided by your inner feeling and allow your hands to go where they intuitively want to during a treatment. It will also usually be right to transfer Reiki at points where the patient feels pain. Therefore, it is not necessary to keep to a rigid system without deviation.

When you start treatment, you should try to give four treatments on four consecutive days at the beginning. These will, above all, stimulate the body to cleanse itself of poisons. The patients should drink a lot of water or tea during this time in order to support the natural detoxication reactions which set in.

First of all, carry out all the basic positions when you give a treatment and leave problematical areas to the end, when they can be treated more intensively. As a rule, each position should be held for three to five minutes. In time you will feel when a zone has received enough Reiki, and you need not keep an eye on the time any more. Problematical areas can be treated for 10 to 20 minutes. Plan enough time for treatment and make sure that it can come to an end harmoniously. A period of at least one hour will generally be necessary. In the case of the old or very ill, treatment should not last longer than 20 to 30 minutes at first, but this can be increased with time if necessary. Ten to 20 minutes will generally be sufficient for small children and infants.

## POINTS TO REMEMBER

- Remove your watch and rings before treatment.
- Wash your hands with water both before and after every treatment.
- The client must take off his shoes and loosen tight clothing such as belt, tie, waistband, brassiere etc. Since Reiki energy will pass through clothing, belts, bandages and plaster casts, other items of clothig need not be removed.
- The client should let his arms lay loosely next to his body. When he is lying on his stomach he can fold them under his head.
- When you lay your hands on the patient, do so gently.
- If the patient's body cannot be touched, as in the case of burns, it will be sufficient to hold your hands a few centimetres above it. (Reiki will work just as effectively up to 2 inches away from the body.)
- Keep your fingers closed during treatment.
- Hold every position for three to five minutes.
- It is very important for the patient not to cross his legs during treatment since this may block the flow of energy.

If you do not feel the familiar warm "flowing" sensation, this does not mean to say that the Reiki energy is not present. It will simply be adapting itself to the needs of the patient.

Ask your patient to take some rest after the treatment. This may be an important time for him, a time when things which came into movement during treatment can continue to pulse and vibrate afterwards with a chance of being resolved. If you feel the wish to express thanks for the Reiki energy you have or are to receive, this can be done before or after treatment.

Reiki helps you or your client to reach a state of optimal health and balance. Above all, never forget, the more Reiki you give, the stronger will be the flow of Reiki energy within you. Energy fills you up before it flows out from your hand. Hence, you also receive a treatment in the process of giving one.

Every healer should chant the following prayer before every healing session:

## REIKI PRAYER

**I thank myself for being here.**
**I thank Reiki for being here.**
**I thank......................for being here.**

**↓**

**(self name (in self-treatment)**
**Patient's name (while treating other)**

# THYMUS GLAND

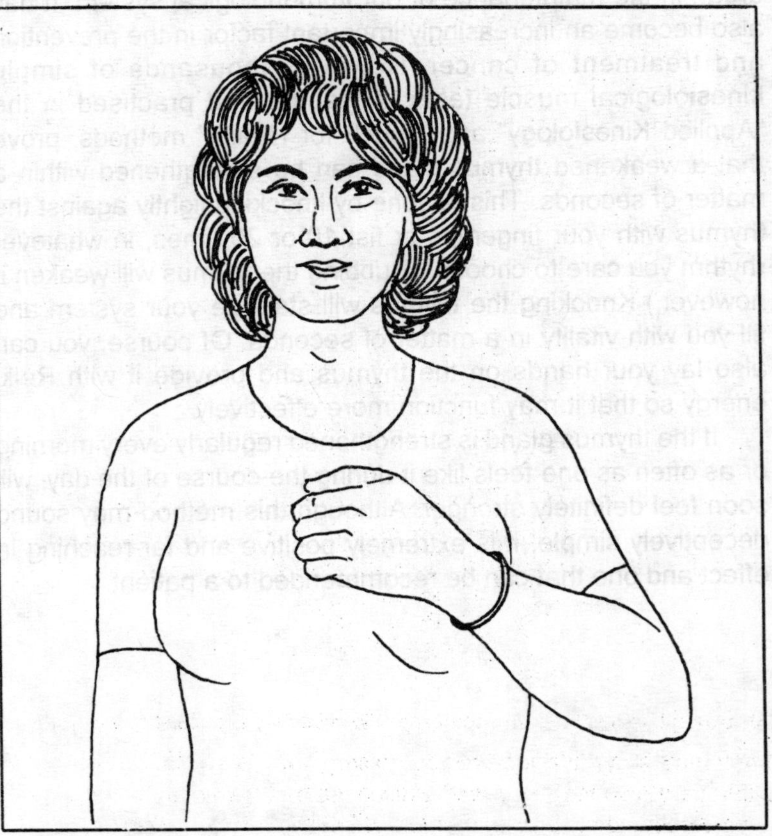

The word "Thymus" is derived from the Greek word *Thymos*, which means life-force or vitality. Here is a simple technique involving the thymus gland which will increase your own inner life-force. Please note, this is not part of the traditional Reiki system of treatment and it is also not taught by Reiki Masters in connection with Reiki either.

It is included here because it is extremely simple and effective. Since it can be combined with Reiki very well it can be included in your programme of treatment.

The thymus gland is situated in the middle of the chest, behind the upper part of the breast-bone. The more we know about the thymus gland, the more significant appears to be its functioning in an overall sense. The thymus is the most important organ in the maintenance of our immunological system. It has also become an increasingly important factor in the prevention and treatment of cancer. However, thousands of simple kinesiological muscle tests, as taught and practised in the "Applied Kinesiology" and "Touch for Health" methods, prove that a weakened thymus gland can be strengthened within a matter of seconds. This is done by knocking lightly against the thymus with your fingertips or fist 10 or 20 times, in whatever rhythm you care to choose. (Rubbing the thymus will weaken it however.) Knocking the thymus will stabilize your system and fill you with vitality in a matter of seconds. Of course, you can also lay your hands on the thymus and provide it with Reiki energy so that it may function more effectively.

If the thymus gland is strengthened regularly every morning or as often as one feels like it during the course of the day, will soon feel definitely stronger. Although this method may sound deceptively simple, it is extremely positive and far-reaching in effect and one that can be recommended to a patient.

# SELF-TREATMENT

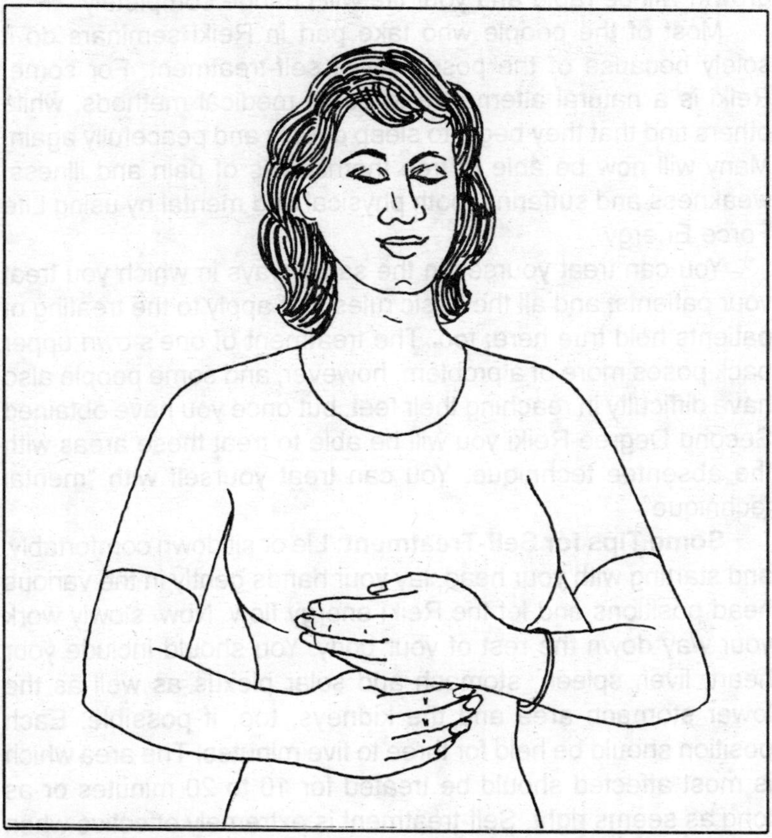

No method of self-treatment can be as simple and as effective as Reiki. You can give yourself treatment whenever you feel like, because Reiki is always with you, and you won't need any special aids or devices either. Whenever you feel pain somewhere, or get into a bad state, when you are tired, worked up or simply scared, you will be able to calm yourself down immediately and relax with your Reiki energy and use it to energize and harmonize yourself.

There is no set rule that you should treat yourself only in unusual situations. Once you have achieved the First Reiki Degree you can energize yourself daily by giving Reiki to yourself. In this way many illnesses will not be able to come near you, and you will be spared much trouble. Your spiritual growth will be rapid and your life will change completely.

Most of the people who take part in Reiki seminars do it solely because of the possibility of self-treatment. For some, Reiki is a natural alternative to usual medical methods, while others find that they begin to sleep deeply and peacefully again. Many will now be able to free themselves of pain and illness, weakness and suffering, both physical and mental by using Life Force Energy.

You can treat yourself in the same ways in which you treat your patients, and all the basic rules that apply to the treating of patients hold true here, too. The treatment of one's own upper back poses more of a problem, however, and some people also have difficulty in reaching their feet, but once you have obtained Second Degree Reiki you will be able to treat these areas with the absentee technique. You can treat yourself with "mental technique".

**Some Tips for Self-Treatment:** Lie or sit down comfortably, and starting with your head, lay your hands gently in the various head positions and let the Reiki energy flow. Now, slowly work your way down the rest of your body. You should include your heart, liver, spleen, stomach and solar plexus as well as the lower stomach area and the kidneys, too, if possible. Each position should be held for three to five minutes. The area which is most affected should be treated for 10 to 20 minutes or as long as seems right. Self-treatment is extremely effective when carried out before falling asleep.

## POINTS TO REMEMBER

- All the following self-treatment positions should be followed daily during cleanse process.
- Self-treatment positions no. 4, 6, 8, 9, 13 and 27 should be followed daily to remain in lush of health.
- Duration of 3 minutes is sufficient for each position.

# SOME SELF-TREATMENT POSITIONS

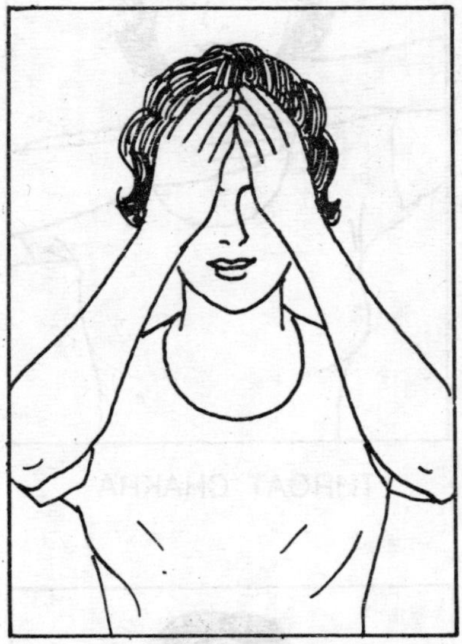

EYES

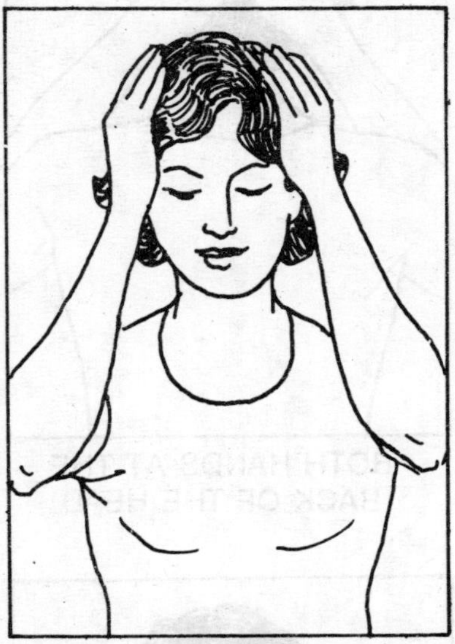

TEMPLES

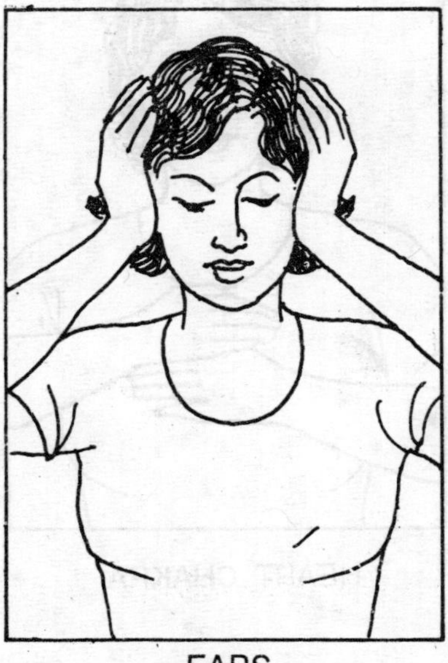

EARS

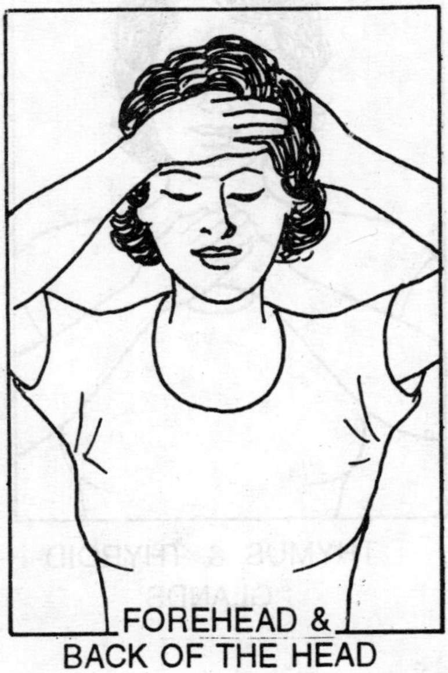

FOREHEAD & BACK OF THE HEAD

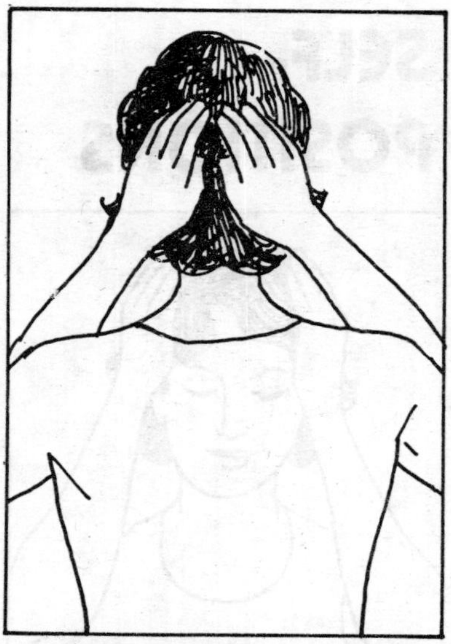

BOTH HANDS AT THE BACK OF THE HEAD

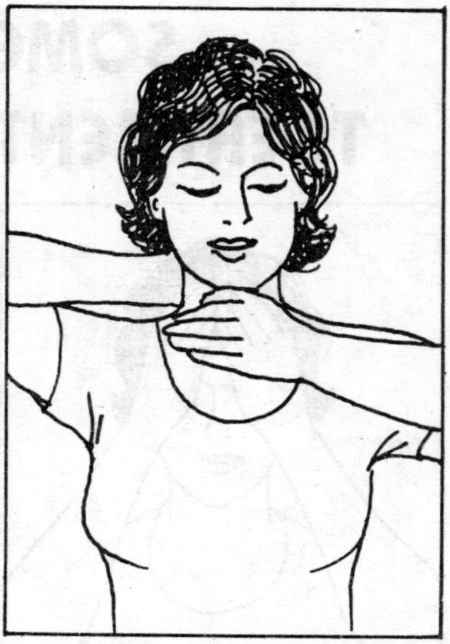

THROAT CHAKRA

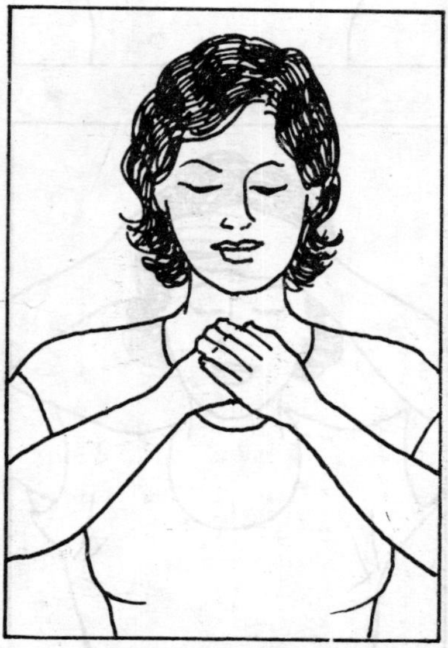

THYMUS & THYROID GLANDS

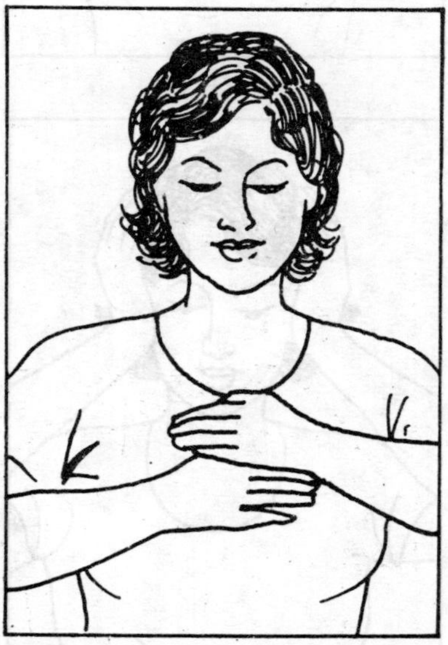

HEART CHAKRA

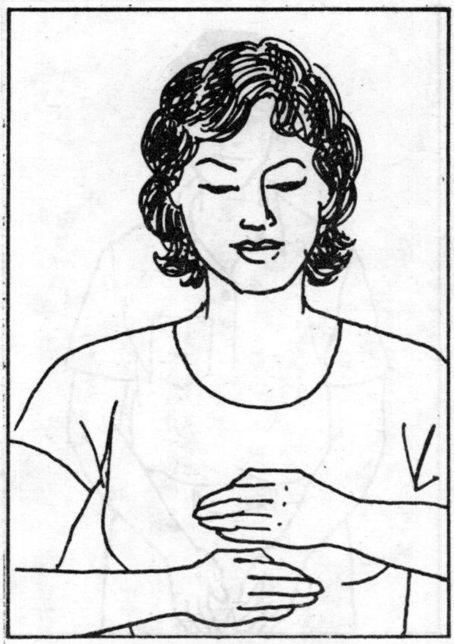

SOLAR PLEXUS

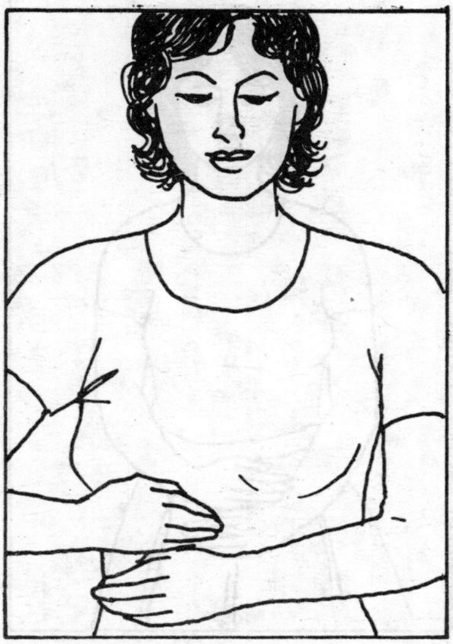

LIVER

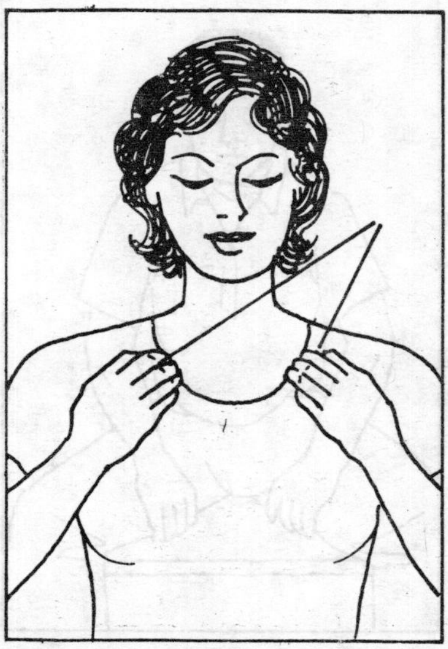

LUNG TIPS

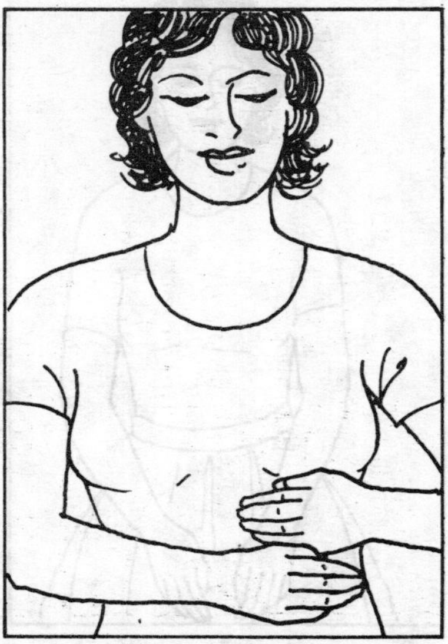

PANCREAS SPLEEN

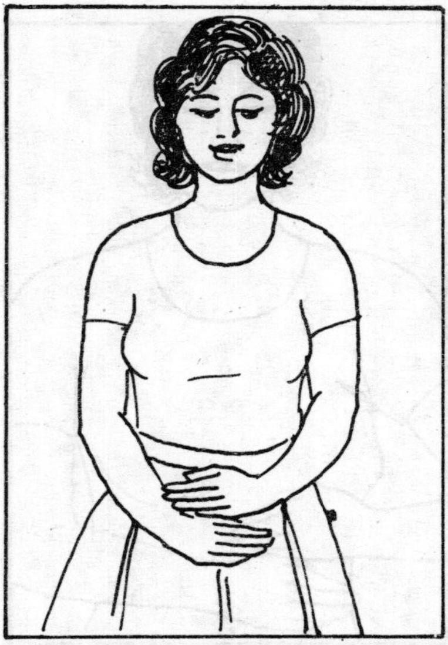

HARA

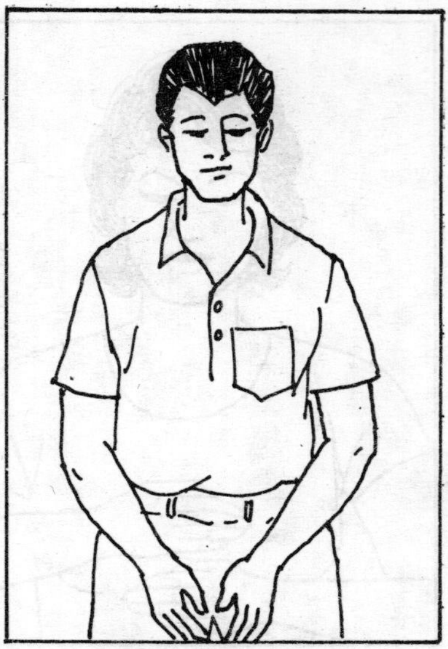

SPERMATIC CORD (GENTS)

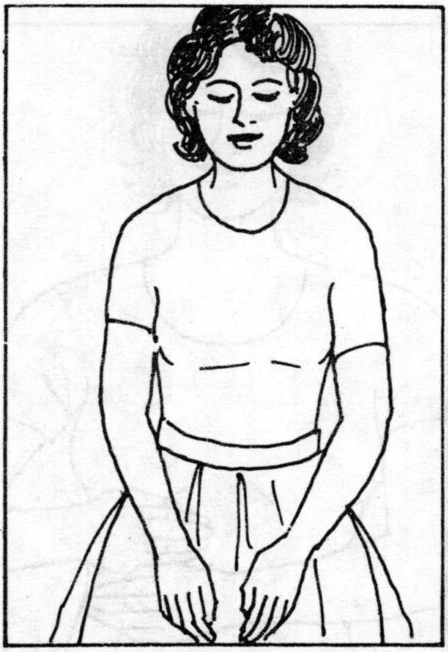

OVARIES (LADIES)

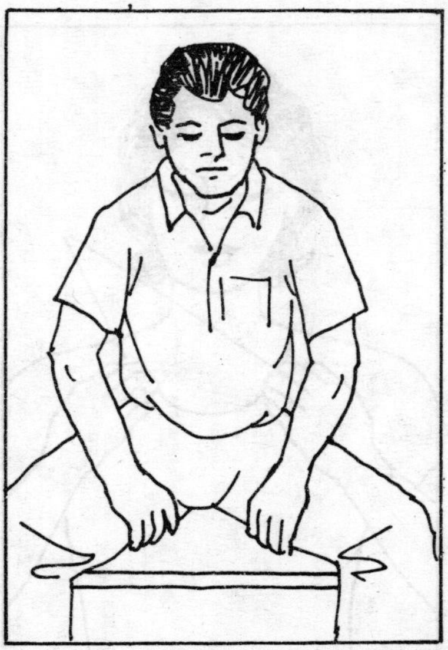

THIGHS

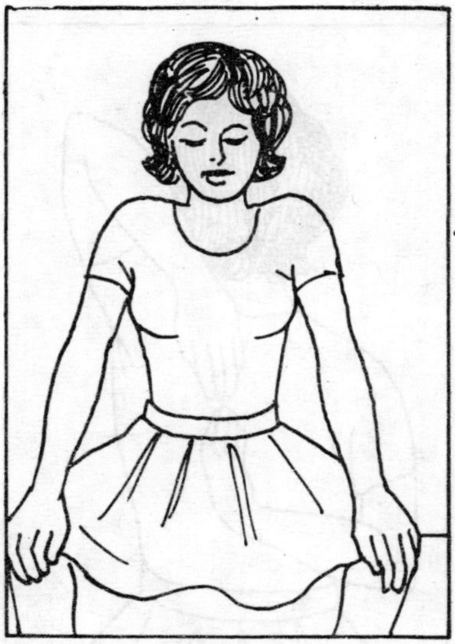

KNEES

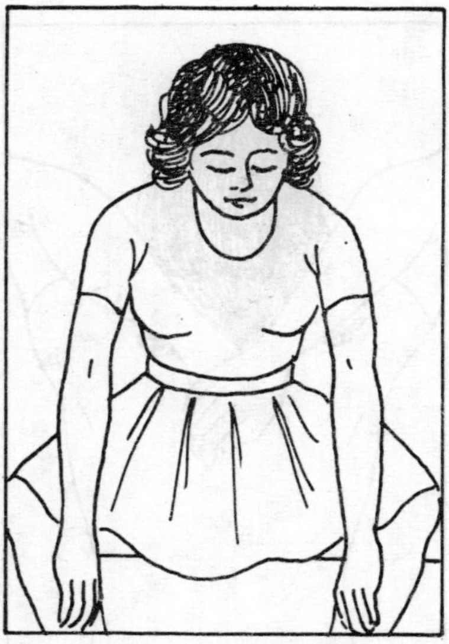

CALF MUSCLES

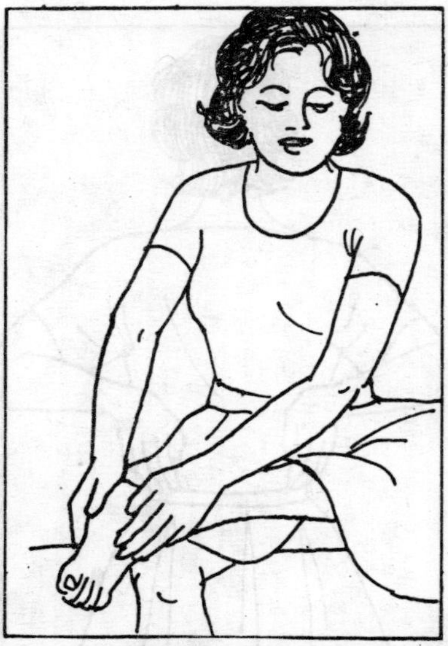

ANKLES & FOOT SOLE

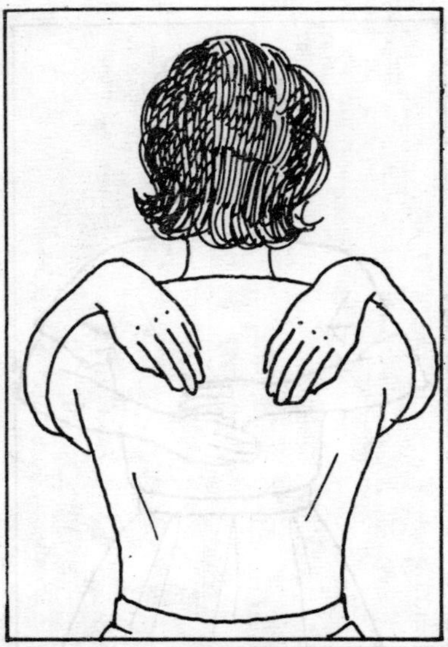

SHOULDERS

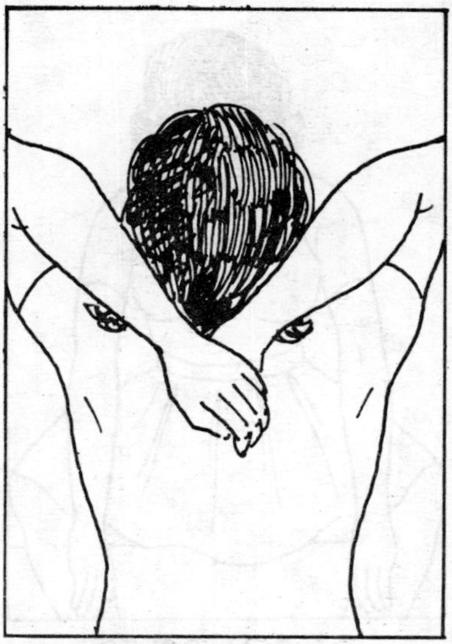

THYMUS & THYROID GLANDS

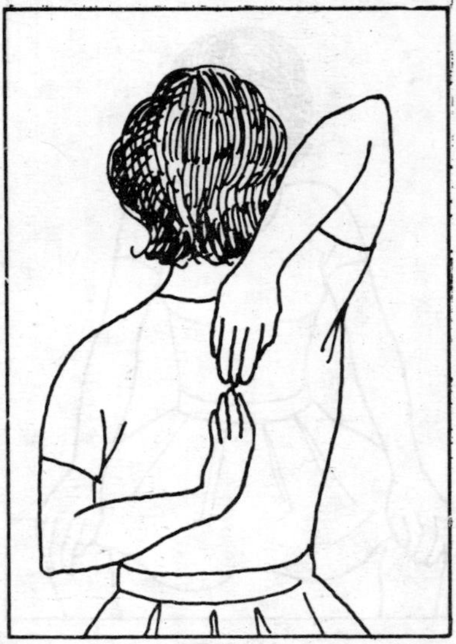

HEART CHAKRA

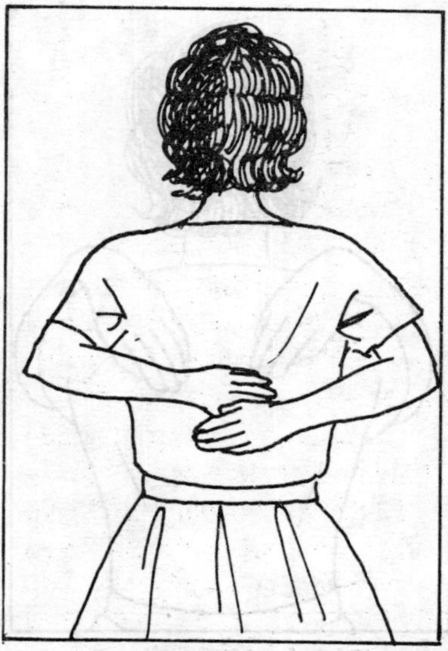

SOLAR PLEXUS

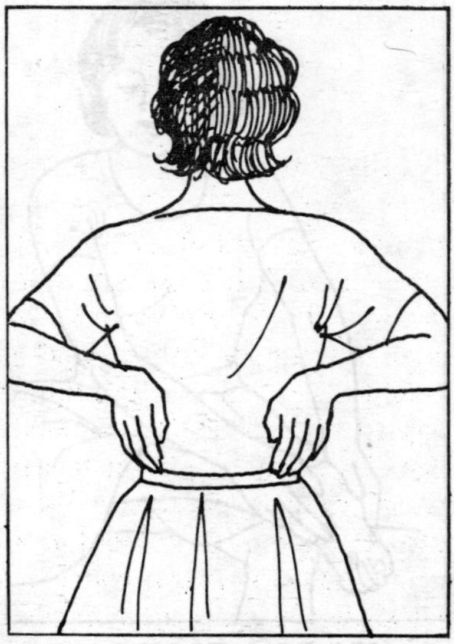

KIDNEYS

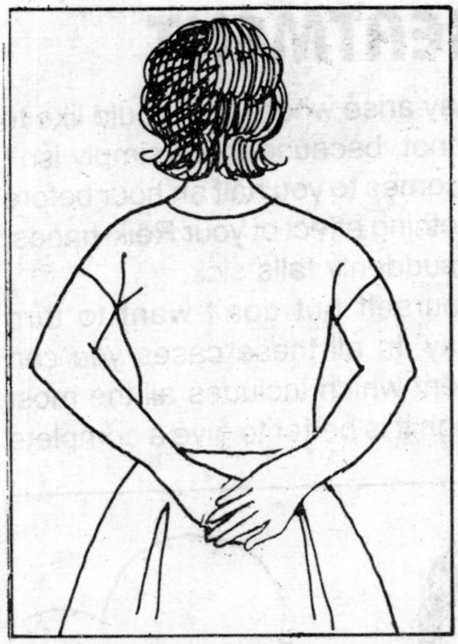

BACK SOLAR PLEXUS

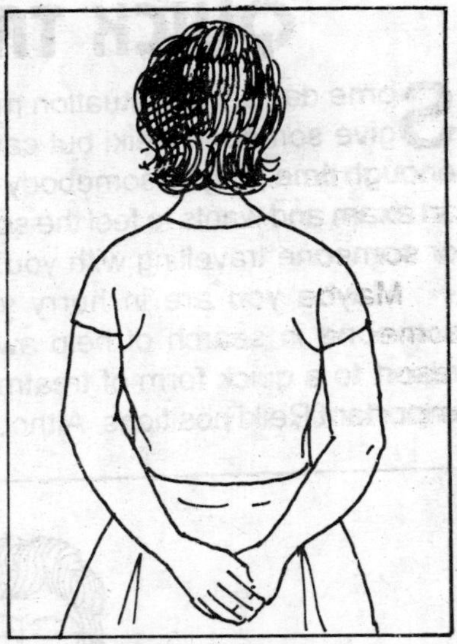

OVER HARA

# QUICK TREATMENT

Some day such a situation may arise where you would like to give someone Reiki but cannot, because there simply isn't enough time. Maybe somebody comes to you half an hour before an exam and wants to feel the soothing effect of your Reiki hands, or someone travelling with you suddenly falls sick.

Maybe you are in hurry yourself but don't want to turn someone in search of help away. In all these cases you can resort to a quick form of treatment which includes all the most important Reiki positions. Although it is better to give a complete

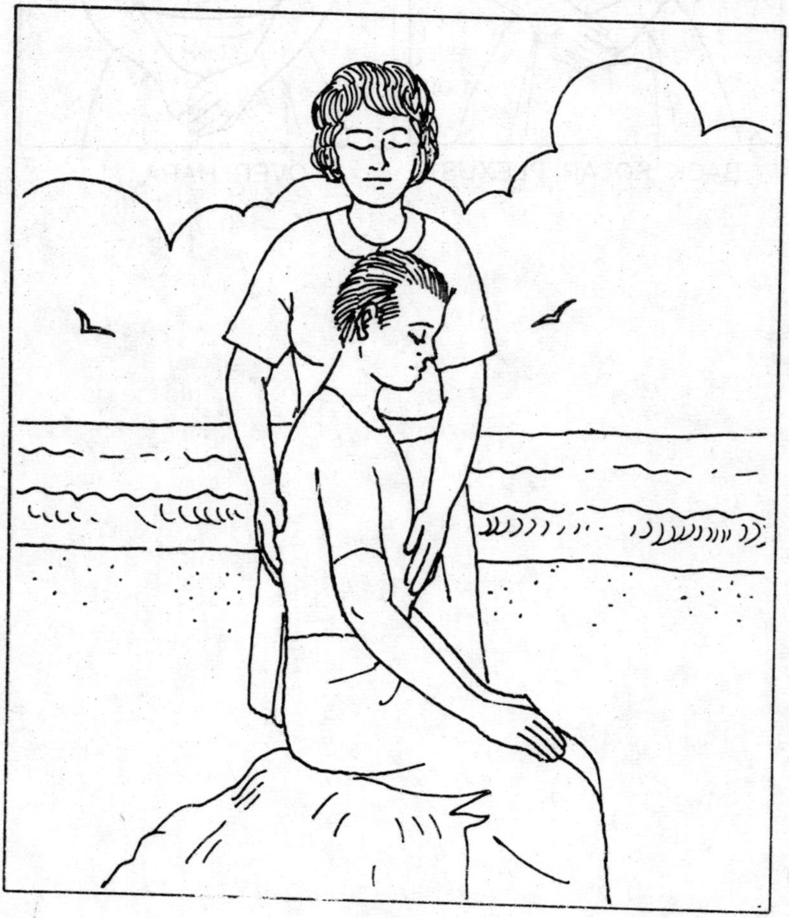

course of treatment, there are times when a short one is better than none at all. However, never give your patient the impression that you are in a hurry. Simply make use of the short time available to you and remain peaceful and tranquil in mood. Even a short treatment can do a miraculous job.

## THE METHODS TO CARRY OUT QUICK TREATMENT

It would be better if patient is sitting on something.

- Lay your hands gently on your patient's shoulders.
- Then gently lay them on the top of his head.
- Lay one hand on the area between the back of the head and the top of the spine, and the other on the forehead.
- Lay one hand on the seventh (protruding) cervical vertibrae and the other in the pit of the throat.
- Lay one hand on the breastbone and the other on the back at the parallel height.
- Lay one hand on the solar plexus and the other at the parallel height on the back.
- Lay one hand on the lower stomach and the other at the bottom of the back at the parallel height.

Reiki is also good as an additional means of giving first aid in the case of accidents and shock. Here you should immediately lay one hand onto the solar plexus and the other onto the kidneys. Once you hav0e done this, move the second hand to the outer edge of the shoulders.

# ABSENTEE HEALING

It will surely surprise many people when they are told that Reiki can be passed on to other people over a long distance. However, in this age, the possibility of this should not surprise or amaze us. For example, we know from radio and television that waves can be sent through the ether and made audible or visible once they have been picked up by the right kind of receiver. We all are familiar with this wireless form of transmission.

Due to the investigation methods developed by modern medical technology, we know today that our brains produce frequencies which differ according to the kind of brain activity causing them. Our thoughts are nothing other than vibratory patterns which are transmitted by our brains, and, like radiowaves, they can be picked up by the right kind of receiver.

We know that not every thought we send out automatically reaches intended recipient and, likewise, it is not sufficient to just send someone Reiki in our thoughts, either. Instead, we have to use a technique which functions as perfectly as calling someone up on the telephone. When we do this, it does not matter that who receives the call. So long as the correct number is dialed, the telephone will ring at the place of right person. This has nothing to do with magic. The laws of physics, which enable us to make telephone calls today were also in existence during ancient times and had simply not yet been discovered and put to use by people of that age.

The natural laws also exist which enable us to transfer Life Force Energy over a long distance, and, even though they have not yet been discovered and confirmed by modern day science, but exist. Moreover, there have always been people who were aware that they existed, people who have developed methods for making successful use of them. The Reiki method of absentee healing is based on these laws and the key to them, which was discovered by Dr Ursui, can be learned in Second Degree Reiki. To keep to our example of the telephone, it is not necessary, however to know all the natural laws responsible for this phenomenon to be able to make use of it for the benefit of mankind.

Absentee healing is needed when you cannot physically be with the person needing treatment, such as someone lying in hospital or living in a far-off place. It is also a method which can immediately be put to use when you are requested for treatment by letter, telephone or telegram.

People who do not know Reiki treatment or never had it at all will be skeptical about absentee healing at first. However, once they have had a normal treatment, they will usually change their attitude to this kind of experiment. Once you have arranged to treat a patient via the absentee method, it will be important to arrange a time when you will both have some peace and quiet. Like direct treatment, absentee healing should be carried out on four successive days. The recipient should not be active during the arranged time but should sit or, it would be better if they would lie down. Make a note of the time arranged and make sure that the recipient knows it, too. In case you do a lot of absentee healing, it will be necessary to plan your appointments conscientiously.

A proper appointment book will help you to avoid an embarrassing situation. Printed appointment cards are also useful, especially when details of your name and address are included, so that the patient can cancel in time, if necessary. Always note the first name and surname of your patients, for you will need these to carry out absentee healing. If the patient is unknown to you, a characteristic photograph of him or her will be necessary, or at least very helpful. This photograph should be with you at the beginning of treatment, complete with details of the full name. However, in urgent cases healer can treat successfully with nothing more than a general description of the person involved and its result would not be discouraging.

After the first three or four successive treatments further ones can then be arranged. A series of treatments can last for several weeks, or even months if necessary. In this case it is best to send Reiki to the recipient at the same time on the same day of the week. This will be convenient for both sides.

Absentee treatment is as good as the direct method, although patients will usually feel the effects of the latter more distinctly

In both cases, the energy will be the same. Many practitioners can feel the flow of Reiki energy in the various parts of the patient's body when they are treating with the absentee method, while others develop a very clear feeling of what is wrong with the patient and what kind of treatment is required.

For absentee healing you do not need a special place, a comfortable place to sit down will be all you need. Also, it does not take up as much time as the "direct" method. Generally 15 to 20 minutes will suffice, although this can vary. Some Reiki Masters also point out that it is possible to treat a large group of people at the same time by applying this method.

It will do no harm for the patient to attune himself to the treatment while it is going on and to let himself flow and be carried along by the stream of energy. You should never carry out an absentee treatment against the will of a person. When two or more practitioners join to send a patient Reiki over a distance, it will be advisable for him to lie down, because the effect can sometimes be powerful.

A man who had requested for Reiki treatment related the following incident: he had made an appointment on telephone with a practitioner for an absentee treatment but when the appointed time came round, he did not pay much attention to the fact and continued to tidy up his garden. He was in the middle of planting seedlings when he suddenly felt an unknown sensation that was so strong he could hardly straighten up. When he later called up his Reiki practitioner, he told him that he had been treating him during this time. This incident impressed him so much that he decided to learn Reiki himself.

One can also treat himself by this method, for example, when you want to treat your back. You do this in exactly the same way as treating someone else over a long distance, and it is a good way of practising the absentee method.

# TOOLS TO USE WITH REIKI

Most of the students, after completing Second Degree, receive very clear intuitive messages to guide them in the healing process. Mrs. Takata herself added a variety of procedures to her treatments, which were not passed down from Usui. Each one of us has our own unique talents, and should feel comfortable about experimenting and even expanding our own repertoire of healing methods. Because Reiki treatment do not require a constant concentration on the channeling of energy to the healee, the healer is left with an opportunity to observe and concentrate his thought processes elsewhere. These tools are not connected directly to Reiki, but you may try some of the following methods with Reiki :

## USE OF SOUND AND COLOUR

The powerful healing effects of colours are widely known.

The qualities of each colour, and their effects on the body are given in following list :

- **Yellow :** Stimulates the digestion, lymphatic system, motor and sensory nerves, and increases hormone production.
- **Orange :** Strengthens lungs and bronchial tubes. Stimulates the thyroid and stomach. Relieves cramps and helps to develop bones.
- **Red :** Energizes the nervous system and stimulates the senses. Activates the circulatory system, gives helping hand to fight infections, heals X-ray damage, and ultra-violet burns.
- **Green :** Balances the cerebrum and physical body, stimulates pituitary and acts as a germicide.
- **Lemon :** Nourishes the brain and body helps clear lungs, stimulates overall body repair.
- **Magenta :** Balances emotions, adjusts blood pressure to perfect balance and stimulates kidneys and adrenals.
- **Scarlet :** Stimulates adrenals and kidneys, reproductive organs and emotions, and raises blood pressure.
- **Blue :** Acts as a sedative, lowers temperature, releaves inflammations, irritations and itching. Also stimulates the pineal gland.

- **Turquoise :** Does repairing job in acute problems, and heals burned skin.
- **Indigo :** Soothes and stimulates parathyroid, shrinks abscesses and tumors, and acts as an emotional depressant.
- **Violet :** Activates spleen and white blood cells, helps reduce temperature, and relaxes muscles.
- **Purple :** Reduces body temperature, rate of heartbeat and blood pressure. Also acts as a kidney depressant, and controls lung haemorrhages.

The students must be encouraged to explore the use of colour, not only in healing but in dress also. Sometimes, while guiding a person through a Reiki/rebirthing session the recipients are encouraged to wear the colour which corresponds to the chakra or energy center where emotional release is needed. The readers would find Jon Monroe's audio colour tapes to be of great help in emotional release work. Jon has made recordings of the twelve sounds or tones which match the twelve colour of Darias Dinshah's vibrational colour scale. The vibrations of colour actually correspond to the different vibrations of certain musical notes. Playing the corresponding chakra colour of an emotionally blocked area of the body, during release work, helps to accelerate healing process.

## CENTERING

In ancient times, millions of physicians and healers were burned as witches and wizards. Actually they were intellectual people of those ages. The irradication of intuitive/psychic abilities began during the dark ages while the religious sanctions against such abilities were promoted to gain further control over the masses by the ruling intellectuals, who used church politics as their weapon. The intellect began to take center stage to the point where today the church has been overshadowed by the hallowed halls of education. Universities, instead of the church, are now the primary conditioning agent for the mass mind/culture. The development of the intellect has reached its height and it has become apparent that it alone cannot provide all of the answers to the massive problems now facing humanity. To help meet the numerous challenges which lie ahead, we must recognize the intellect's true places as a tool, and not continue to identify with it as the essence of who we are. The next step that we must take is to redevelop our latent intuitive abilities like people of dark ages.

The attunements of First and Second Degree Reiki helps to open up intuitive knowledge. Continued self-treatments also help to further development of this quality. In Reiki classes, teachers teach a very simple process to their students, to help them focus their consciousness in their hara or feeling center of their bodies. When we are centered in the hara or chi center, as the Chinese call the emotional/sexual chakra (spleen chakra), the opposite polarity chakra located in the third eye also becomes balanced and opens up. By literally sidelining the intellect and bringing the center of our attention (the focus of our conscious awareness), into the "belly" chakra, we begin to connect with our true feelings. Once we are centered in the hara, we naturally open up to the intuitive faculties located in the third eye chakra.

In this process the students are asked to sit in a comfortable position either on the floor in lotus position with legs folded and back slightly forward, or in a chair (also leaning forward so that the spine is perfectly balanced and relaxed) with the ears over the shoulders and the shoulders over the hips. Reiki Master then begin to lead them through the visualization.

## EXERCISE

Please note that most of the healers follow this particular exercise :

- Begin by taking nice long slow deep breaths.
- Inhale through the mouth and exhale through the nose.
- Just keep on breathing—nice long slow, deep breaths.
- Visualize a beautiful golden ball floating just above the top of your head. This ball is the glowing ball of your conscious awareness.
- Continue to breathe.
- See your breath expanding the golden glowing ball of your consciousness. Each time you exhale, the beautiful golden sparkling light of your consciousness emanates outward.
- Continue breathing nice long slow deep breaths.
- Take one more deep breath into the golden ball of your consciousness. When you exhale, begin to see the golden

ball float gently down through the top of your head and begin to blend with the lovely purple glowing ball of the Crown Chakra.

- Take another deep breath into the now golden purple glowing light of your spiritual consciousness.
- Watch as it expands with your breath, filling with warmth and light and as you begin to exhale, see the light emanate and sparkle outward, sending the beautiful light of your consciousness to those around you.
- Continue to take nice long slow deep breaths into the golden purple ball. See it expand again with your breath, and then, as you exhale see the beautiful sparkling light glowing, radiating outward.
- Continue to breathe long slow deep breaths.
- Inhale slowly, as you begin to exhale, see the golden ball gently separate from the purple center of your spiritual consciousness and float slowly downward to the center right behind your brow, the beautiful indigo glowing center of intuition.
- Notice the golden ball as it melts and become one with the beautiful glowing ball of your intuitive knowingness.
- Continue to breathe.

  Take another deep breath into the now golden indigo ball, filling it with the warmth and light of the breath.

  And then, as you exhale, see the beautiful golden indigo light permeating the air around you.
- Take a nice long slow deep breath into the golden indigo ball. Feel the breath filling it with the light of your intuitive consciousness and then sparkling and flowing out into the surrounding environment.
- Continue to breathe.
- Take one more nice long slow deep breath into the golden indigo chakra.
- As you exhale, see the golden ball begin to gently separate from the indigo glowing chakra and descend slowly down towards the throat into the lovely light blue turquoise glowing chakra. See the two become one, filling your communication center with the energy of your breath.

- And as you exhale, send the light and love from your communication center out towards those around you.
- Keep on breathing nice long slow deep breaths.
- As you inhale, see the golden turquoise ball fill with the light and energy of your breath.
- As you exhale, see the turquoise-golden light emanate and sparkle out toward those around you.
- Now begin to take one more nice long slow deep breath into the turquoise-golden ball.
- As you exhale, see the golden ball again begin to separate and float slowly and gently down into the heart center, the lovely emerald glowing center of your heart.
- See the golden ball begin to merge with the lovely emerald green ball, filling your heart with the consciousness of your love.
- Continue breathing as you inhale. Feel the breath fill your heart with the light and energy of love.
- And then slowly, as you begin to exhale, see the beautiful emerald-gold light sparkling and radiating the energy of your love to all of those around you.
- See it continuing out in waves, washing over the planet filling it with love.
- And then, as you inhale again, feel the energy of love returning with your breath as it fills you and expands you with the emerald-golden glowing light of the heart center.
- Take one more long deep breath into the emerald-golden ball, again filling it with the light of love, as you exhale.
- Begin to see the golden ball of your consciousness begin to separate and float slowly down into the solar plexus—your center of power and wisdom.
- See the golden light merge and become one with the brilliant yellow glowing ball of the solar plexus right between the rib cage.
- Continue to take nice long slow deep breaths.
- See your breath expanding the now golden-yellow ball with the energy of your wisdom and power center, filling it with the power of love and gratitude.
- As you exhale, see the light sparkling and sending out its rays of power to those around you.

- Take another deep breath, again filling the golden-yellow center with the energy of your breath.
- And as you exhale, feel the light and warmth of your power and wisdom radiating outward and filling each person with the empowerment of love.
- Take one more nice long slow deep breath into the golden yellow chakra.
- Now, as you exhale, see the golden ball slowly begin to separate and float gently down into the lovely orange chakra, three finger widths below the navel, filling the ki or chi center with the golden light of your consciousness.
- With each warm breath, feel your belly filling with the golden-orange light of your emotional/sexual center.
- And as you exhale, feel the emotions of love sparkle their lovely golden-orange light to all around you.
- Continue to breathe nice long slow deep breaths, filling the belly with the emotions of love, and again sending the golden-orange light outward to those around you.
- Just keep on breathing into the belly, filling it with the consciousness of your love, feel the warm glow of the orange-golden light as your consciousness rests in your center. Feel the peace and tranquility.
- Continue to breathe.
- Take one more long slow deep breath in the hara.
- And as you exhale, see the golden light begin to slip away and again float gently downward towards the tip of the sacrum, down into the red Root Chakra. As the two merge and become, one, feel the heat of the beautiful golden-red light begin to fill the entire pelvic area, filling it with the light of love and abundance.
- As you inhale, feel the golden-red light fill the pelvic area with the consciousness of love, transmuting all of the survival issues of this chakra with the energy of abundance.
- As you exhale, see the beautiful golden-red light sparkle and emanate towards those around you, sending your abundance outward in waves of light.
- And then, as you inhale, feel this light returning and filling you again with an overflowing of abundance.
- Just keep on breathing.

- With each breath you feel the energy of prosperity and abundance fill your entire body, starting in the Root Chakra and radiating out from there, continuing to fill the entire body.
- As you exhale, see the light and love of abundance flowing out around you.
- The next time you inhale, see the golden ball gently separate from the red Root Chakra and float gently upward, back towards the hara, returning to the beautiful orange glowing light of your feeling center.
- As you exhale, see the orange and golden light become one.
- Continue to breathe nice long slow deep breaths into your center, feeling very tranquil and totally at peace.
- As you inhale, the orange-golden light fills your entire being with the emotion of love.
- As you exhale, feel all disruptive emotions fading away. Each time you inhale, you feel more fully grounded and at center, flooding your belly with the love energy of your breath.
- As you exhale again, see the orange-golden light of your love energy streaming out, overflowing with the abundance of your love; and then, with the in breath, flowing back to you with the same waves of love and abundance. Contemplate the peace and calm in your center, and then open channel. This makes you feel at one with all those around you, and with your environment.
- As you relax in this calm center, slowly begin to open your eyes and again become aware of your environment. It would be more convenient if you would record the whole process and play back to yourself.

The above mentioned exercise is designed to help you develop the feeling of being centered. As you move progressively through each chakra, you may occasionally feel resistance at specific chakras to the movement of your consciousness between them. If you feel blocked in any area as you follow this procedure, you can exhale several times in an abrupt and powerful manner to help "blow out" any clogged areas. Once you develop the feeling of being centered, you can shorten this exercise by exhaling two or three times within seconds bringing the center of your consciousness quickly down into the belly. as you allow your intellect to step aside, and at the same time, put yourself into an alpha state, two of the benefits inherent in this exercise.

The successful healers seem to work in an alpha state, which in turn, the healee seems to pick up by "osmosis" during the healing. The students should be asked to walk into a crowded area or market alive with noises, and take a few moments to become deeply centered. It is amazing how quickly the area around you grows calm and peaceful, and the conversation often recedes to a tranquil murmur. It is important to note that when this occurs, it is not you who is affecting the people, it is simply that the alpha state is absorbed automatically by those around us. In other words, if someone is in alpha state, he acts as a natural channel for the energy to be transmitted to others who are close to him.

Making an effort to center oneself on a daily basis is a certain way to maintain a more tranquil lifestyle. It not only will help to keep one in a state of emotional balance and health, but it may even permeate the energy fields of those around him without any real effort, and transmit the same Life Force Energy.

# THE CHAKRAS

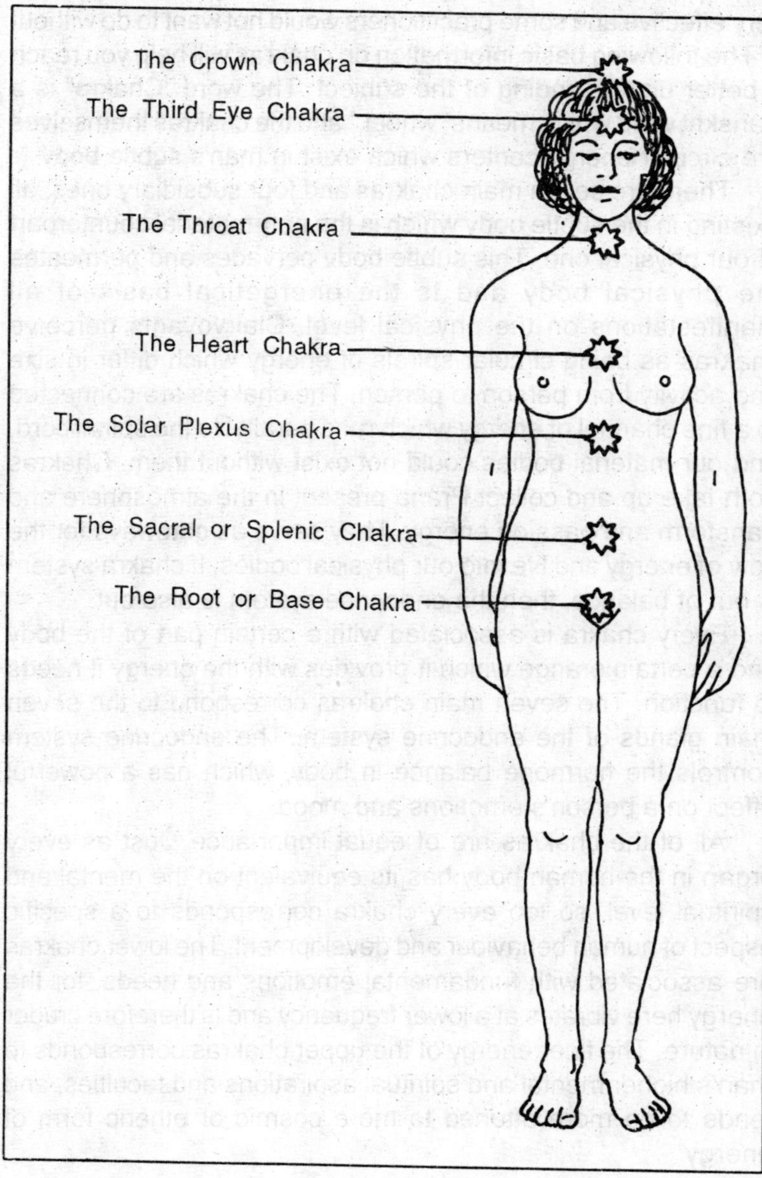
The Crown Chakra
The Third Eye Chakra
The Throat Chakra
The Heart Chakra
The Solar Plexus Chakra
The Sacral or Splenic Chakra
The Root or Base Chakra

The location of the *chakras* in the etheric body corresponds directly to the placement of the endocrine gland in the physical body. Balancing out the chakras with the help of Reiki is not part of the usual programme of treatment. However, it is very effective and some practitioners would not want to do without it. The following basic information on chakras will help you reach a better understanding of the subject. The word "Chakra" is a Sanskrit word which means "wheel," and the chakras themselves are circular energy centers which exist in man's subtle body.

There are seven main chakras and four subsidiary ones, all existing in the subtle body which is the non-material counterpart of our physical one. This subtle body pervades and permeates the physical body and is the energetical basis of all manifestations on the physical level. Clairvoyants perceive chakras as being circular spirals of energy which differ in size and activity from person to person. The chakras are connected to a fine channel of energy which runs parallel to the spinal cord, and our material bodies could not exist without them. Chakras both take up and collect Prana present in the atmosphere and transform and pass on energy. They serve as gateways for the flow of energy and life into our physical bodies. If chakra system is out of balance, then the endocrine system is also out.

Every chakra is associated with a certain part of the body and a certain orange which it provides with the energy it needs to function. The seven main chakras correspond to the seven main glands of the endocrine system. The endocrine system controls the hormone balance in body, which has a powerful effect on a person's emotions and mood.

All of the chakras are of equal importance. Just as every organ in the human body has its equivalent on the mental and spiritual level, so too every chakra corresponds to a specific aspect of human behaviour and development. The lower chakras are associated with fundamental emotions and needs, for the energy here vibrates at a lower frequency and is therefore cruder in nature. The finer energy of the upper chakras corresponds to man's higher mental and spiritual aspirations and faculties, and tends to be more attuned to more cosmic or etheric form of energy.

Any kind of blockage in the energy flow of the chakras as well as an excess of energy can lead to imbalance and disharmony on the physical, mental and spiritual levels. Such disturbances are often caused by psychological stress and trauma as well as by painful experiences of excitement.

These chakras have fine antennae which react to every influence coming from outside and which can open up or draw together accordingly. For this reason, the individual chakras in most people vibrate at different frequencies. In normal, undisturbed conditions, the chakras harmonize. A healer can do a lot by simply "purifying" the chakras and balancing them out so that the energy flows again without disturbance. All meditation and yoga systems seek to balance out the energy of the chakras by purifying the lower energies and guiding them upwards. If one chakra is out of balance then the function associated with it also get out of balance.

## SEVEN MAIN CHAKRAS

***The Crown Chakra*** is positioned at the top of the head, at the fontanel. This chakra represents the highest level of consciousness that mankind can attain, known as enlightenment. In a nutshell, it connects us with our spiritual self. (For this reason a spiritually awakened person is often represented with a halo or rays of light around his head.) This chakra is the seat of intuition and direct spiritual vision.

***Gland :*** the pineal gland (the epiphysis).

***Organs :*** the upper brain and the right eye situated in the middle of the forehead, a little higher than the eyebrows. It is the center of such forms of extrasensory perception such as clairvoyance and telepathy. It is the seat of the will, the intellect and the spirit; it is here that we visualize things. The opening of the Third Eye corresponds to spiritual awakening.

***Gland :*** the pituitary gland (the hypohysis).

***Organs :*** the spine, tne lower brain, the left eye, the nose and the ears.

**The Throat Chakra** is also known as the Thyroid or Laryngeal Chakra. It is the chakra of communication, self-expression and creativity. This is where you hear your inner voice and ones coming from extrasensory realms.

***Gland :*** the thyroid gland.

***Organs :*** the throat, upper lungs, digestive tract and arms.

***The Heart Chakra*** is positioned in the middle of the chest at the height of the heart. It is the center of real, unconditional affection as well as spiritual growth, compassion, brotherliness, devotion and love. Many eastern methods of meditation are especially designed to open up this chakra.

***Gland :*** the thymus.

***Organs :*** the heart, the liver, the lungs and circulatory system.

**The Solar Plexus Chakra** lies slightly above the navel. It is the actual center of the body, the place where physical energy is distributed. It is also the center of unrefined emotions and the power urge. When we are scared, we can feel this area tightening up. In a nutshell it is the power and wisdom center.

***Gland :*** the pancreas.

***Organs :*** the stomach, liver and gall-bladder (digestive system).

***The Sacral or Splenic Chakra*** is positioned slightly below the navel, in front of the sacrum. It is the center of sexual energy (both as transmitter and receiver) and of the ego. The feelings of other people are directly perceived with this chakra, making it one of the centers of extrasensory perception.

***Glands:*** the gonads.

***Organs :*** the reproductive organs and the legs.

**The Root or Base Chakra** lies in the area of the coccyx in men and between the ovaries in women. This chakra is the seat of physical vitality and the fundamental urge to survive. It regulates those mechanisms which keep the physical body alive. Seat of kundalini, creative expression, abundance issues.

***Glands :*** the suprarenal glands.

***Organs :*** the kidneys, the bladder and the spine.

In order to balance the *chakras* with the help of Reiki, a deeper knowledge of the way they function will not necessarily be required, for the energy of Reiki functions in its own, optimal way. It is therefore very easy to practise this form of Reiki. You can balance out the energy of the chakras by laying your hands on each of them successively, beginning with the Third Eye Chakras for example and working your way down to the Root

Chakra or vice versa. A further possibility would be to lay one hand on the Third Eye Chakra and the other on the Root Chakra and then to move your hands to the Throat Chakra and the Sacral Chakra, the Heart Chakra and the Solar Plexus Chakra successively. Be sure to engage your intuitive knowingness when balancing bodily energies. Always leave your hands in position until you can feel the same amount or kind of energy flowing through them. For people who do too much mental labour, you can lay one hand on the Third Eye Chakra and, leaving it there, move your other hand from one lower chakra to the other, beginning with the Root Chakra, to balance them out. Do not touch the Crown Chakra, or the Lotus Chakra, when doing this form of treatment, since the highest state of consciousness requires neither harmonization nor the provision of additional energy. Feel free to connect different combination of chakras, because each person has different imbalances, and a different combination may suit to his need.

After obtaining Second Degree Reiki you will also be able to treat the chakras with the symbols you have learned. They can also be treated with the mental and absentee methods.

Once the chakras are balanced, they will automatically create balance in all of the systems of the body and dissolve blockages of energy and set potential capabilities free. Make use of this special form of Reiki treatment whenver the need arises.

## CRYSTALS

People consider working with crystals to be a very modern phenomenon, but crystals are used since ages. Quartz Crystal has become very popular in recent years as a tool which helps to amplify and direct the natural energies of the healer. With the quantum leap taking place in man's consciousness, some of what is thought to be ancient Atlantean crystal technology is now coming to light. In addition to the exploration of crystal healing methods, which are being conducted by many individuals, traditional science has also discovered the powerful properties of the crystalline structure. In recent years, science has begun to utilize crystal technology for solar power, communications, and information storage. The piezo-electric effect, which occurs when crystals are placed under pressure, and as a result, emit measurable electrical voltage, is one property which is now being utilized. In other words, by mechanically squeezing a quartz crystal, it begins to emit electrons. Conversely, applying an electrical current to a crystal causes mechanical movement. The regularity at which the mechanical movement occurs is quite precise, which is the reason why quartz crystals are so useful in keeping time. Each crystal gives off its own energy based on its colour, clarity, cut, size, hardness, etc.

Crystals are nature's product, but now the science has developed the technology to grow them synthetically. A crystal is a geometrically formed fused mineral, sugar or substance, whose molecules or atoms are arranged in a repeating pattern, which gives the external shape a symmetrical appearance. The stable geometrical/mathematical orderliness which crystals maintain with extreme precision is also a clue to their usefulness as a programming tool. Their capacity to form and hold a specific energy matrix and transduce information between the subtle levels or planes of existence is another factor behind their usefulness.

Wearing gemstones, in form of jewellery, brings the energy of the stone into one's auric field. Whereas Reiki energy penetrates the physical and etheric bodies simultaneously, as well as, penetrating the mental level where the causal factor of disease lies, crystals seem to work primarily on the subtle energetic bodies. As has been previously mentioned, disruptive patterns in the etheric body can often be seen by clairvoyants and registered by sensitive instruments before they manifest at the physical level in the form of disease. Herein lies the inherent usefulness of crystals, which is to amplify and focus energy directly at specific areas of blockage in the etheric system. If disease is already manifest in the physical system, the positive changes that crystals help to make on the etheric level will eventually also effect correction on the physical level. Thus crystals are a great help in removing energy blocks and negative thought forms on the subtle energetic level, but they will not necessarily be able to release a long ingrained mental or emotional pattern which lies at the causal level of disease. From the above information it can be seen that crystals provide us with a powerful tool to amplify and direct healing energy, but they cannot prevent the healee from recreating the negative thought form which makes way for the illness.

Like other healing modalities, there are also many ways that crystals may be used with Reiki to promote further healing. While Second Degree Reiki offers a complete system for absentee healing, the First Degree student can program a crystal with Reiki by holding it between the hands and charging it with Life Force Energy.

Then crystal may be given as loan or presented to someone who needs healing so that they may treat themselves or carry it on their body. Crystals can be charged with a healing thought form which is sent out over a distance by holding the crystal and visualizing the energy being received by the healee. As crystals operate at the level of magnetoelectric frequencies, the mind-directed energies of the sender are amplified and simultaneously transmitted from a distance to the healee. The Second Degree student can further programme a crystal with the special mental healing techniques to further amplify the energies needed to effect change on the causal level. Such a process using the Second Degree level helps to further activate the crystal to higher levels of vibratory frequency.

Crystal charging means the renewal of a crystal's vibrational charge whereas activation increases it's overall charge capacity. It has been observed that the First Degree Reiki charges a crystal, and Second Degree tends to actually activate a crystal by increasing its overall charge capacity.

## Selection of Crystal

Before choosing a crystal it is important to find which one resonates with your energy field. Just as people have different energy patterns, crystals also have their own unique vibrations. The colour, size, shape, and type are all important factors in crystal selection, along with the intended use. Your best guide is your intuition, and your own sensitivity to the subtle energy field coming from the crystal.

## Exercise to Develop Sensitivity to Subtle Energies

- Rub your palms together briskly for about one minute.
- Move your hands (palms facing each other) slowly apart until they are around six inches apart, then slowly move them towards each other until they almost touch. Continue doing this as you try to feel any tingling sensations, heat changes, or any other subtle energy change in your hands. Once you have developed this sensitivity, try moving your hands over the top of a group of crystals, to feel same kind of energy.

## Cleansing and Clearing Crystals

After obtaining a crystal, it is better to clear it, as quartz crystal tends to absorb any vibrations which are (or have been) in its close vicinity. Crystals tend to absorb and store the energy and thought patterns of people who have held them or been in close contact with them. Crystals which are worn or used daily should be cleansed on a regular basis (at least once a week). Those which are generally kept in a harmonious environment need only periodic cleansings. Some of the various methods for clearing crystals are, soaking them in a salt water solution for at least twenty-four hours, placing and covering them in dry sea salt for at least twenty-four hours, cleansing them with running water, and also by blowing on each of their facets while visualizing them becoming pure and clean.

## Crystal Charging

To renew the vibrational charge of a crystal, several methods may be used. You can put the crystal in the center of a crystal gridwork or under a pyramid for a number of hours. Surrounding crystals with colour gels and projecting light is one way to charge them with the different vibratory rates of colour. Also, leaving crystals in a highly energized point on the earth, such as in vortex area or one with a low geomagnetic pressure, will help to give a charge. Finally, Reiki is a very powerful tool for charging crystals. Charging can be accomplished by any Reiki practitioner who holds a crystal between their hands, with the intention of charging it, and then focusing on the purpose for which they intend to use it.

## How to Activate Crystal

The activation of a crystal means expanding its overall energy capacity so that it may accept a greater charge. Some experts recommend exposing a crystal to high and very low temperatures to induce activation. However, the temperature changes must be gradual to prevent any cracking of the crystal. Exposing them to extreme weather conditions such as lightning, storms, blizzards, are also recommended, along with the use of Tesla coils, electrostatic generators, and even more elaborate crystal gridworks. Second Degree Reiki can also be applied to increase crystal capacity.

## Crystal Programming

Like science which now uses crystal technology to store memory in computers, the individual can learn to program quartz crystals for many different purposes. Programming is essentially the process of storing specific energy and thought patterns in a crystal. Here are two examples of crystal programming :

**Healing:** Crystal can also be programmed for specific health problems. Visualize the person's health problems or any kind of problem getting better, feel the healing energy flowing into the crystal, visualize the problem completely healed. Be as detailed as possible. After the programming process, you can give the person a treatment by holding the crystal over his body and guide the energy where you want it with your mind. Visualize the energy flowing from you through the crystal and into the person's body. You can also give or loan the crystal to the persons to treat themselves or just carry it with them. After a few treatments it is advisable to cleanse and reprogram the crystal for further use.

**Colour Programming** : Every colour has a certain vibrational quality that can be used for numerous purposes. Colour can be used to induce changes in personality, emotions, states of mind and physical disorders. The colour for the change that you desire is programmed into the crystal and used in the same manner as above. Coloured plastic gels can be put around the crystal and placed in front of a light source (sunlight in front of lamp, light box, etc.) to accelerate the programming process.

Remember that crystals are neutral objects which emit energy, and extend and amplify their programs in a coherent, highly concentrated form. As previously mentioned, programming is the process of storing specific energy and thought patterns so that they may then be transmitted into objects of people at will. It is important to note that anyone choosing to work with crystals should exercise responsibility, because, although they may be used for mind to mind communication, their purpose, best is in the service of humanity for the removal of pain and suffering. For those who are acquainted with the history of Atlantis, whether you take it as fact or myth, it stands as a powerful example of the need to take caution and exercise increased individual and collective responsibility for the higher levels of technology which are currently being developed. Crystals can be programmed as powerful tools to help the individual promote further self-transformation. When used with Reiki they do a wonderful job.

## REMOVAL OF ENERGY BLOCKS

Sometimes it is observed that a particular area of the body seems to draw very little or no energy and perhaps even feels cold to the touch. When you are quite sure that you are feeling an energy block, and that your hands do not feel cool because they are drawing enough energy to feel hot in comparison to the patient's body temperature, you may choose to utilize the following technique : After having laid your hands on a very cool area of the body for five to ten minutes, without any sensation of energy being drawn in a quicker fashion, you may intuitively sense that an energy block is present. In order to remove it, you can scoop the energy into a tight compressed ball at the surface of the skin, grasp it with your left hand, and lift it away from the body. Sever it with your right hand by making a slicing motion next to the surface of the skin, and then lift the right hand to the left using it to surround the left in white light, and let the ball of energy go. When you return your hands to the body, you will generally feel a definite increase in the flow of energy, because the person is wide open to receive the Life Force Energy.

One thing to keep in your mind about this procedure is that it is possible to do it entirely in the mind's eye. In other words, there are times when the personality or belief system of the patient is such that to move the hands as described, would seem like a foolish thing to him. On the other hand, there are times when certain people would benefit by visually seeing you extract the energy as verification that something negative has indeed been removed.

Sometimes people are aware, on a subconscious level, of an energy block in the body. Sometimes dramatizing the actual removal of these same blocks helps to convince the conscious mind of the healee that a change has indeed taken place, and thus accelerates the healing. Often the person will experience the movement of energy in the body or heat during the procedure. Reiki itself is very powerful and will gradually diffuse most energy blocks in time. However, using such a conscious process as described above helps to remove blocks more quickly and effectively.

There are various ways which can create energy blocks. For the most part, they are a result of stored emotions which have not been able to be expressed. A chapter on Body Psychology is already given in this book, it gives an indepth look at the various causes of emotional blocks, and in particular, which types of emotions are stored in specific areas of the body. Another cause of energy blocks is due to negative thoughts, which when a person becomes obsessed with them, seem to take on an energy or life force of their own. These may eventually attach themselves to the body in a large mass.

You must be aware of this fact that our thoughts are indeed very powerful. All of our thoughts amass in the etheric or energy body of the earth, which is why it is so important that we become consciously aware individuals. Thoughts which pass through us quickly do not generally take on a life force of their own, and are soon dissipated. However, if a person becomes obsessed with a negative idea over a period of time, the force of these thoughts will create actual "little beings" called elementals, which will in turn help perpetuate the same thoughts. Long standing feuds are powerful examples of the life force in elementals. On the other hand, positive thoughts which are repeated over and over also create a life force of their own, and will perpetuate themselves. It is very important for people to understand this phenomenon, because at the present time, with the powerful love energy entering the earth to create healing, many people are experiencing large awakenings which are affecting their intuitive faculties. Some are even developing the ability to see elementals, and beginning to think that they are losing their minds, due to the lack of cultural references to explain such happenings.

In western society there is still great fear about psychic abilities. This is largely due to the centuries of witch trials, in which millions of intellectuals who were practicing medicine and spiritual healing were burned and tortured, that resulted in the demise of the intuitive faculty, and the development of logic and rationalization which reached its height under the reign of such thinkers as Descartes. In our world, rationalization and logic have come to dominate thinking, but it is plain to see that it does not solve all of our problems. Today we see a blend occurring as the intellect begins to take its proper place beside the intuitive faculty and is relegated to its proper place as a tool of the mind. As we begin to develop greater ability in the intutive realm, some of the very ancient and very normal human psychic abilities are returning. We are all naturally telepathic. It is clear that even animals have these abilities; that indeed they think in pictures as has been shown by certain psychics reading the minds of sick animals, to help aid veterinarians in diagnosing their illnesses. If animals have these abilities, then why should not humans? More and more people are developing greater intuitive abilities, especially after receiving Second Degree Reiki. People must realize that these are God-gifted qualities.

If people experience psychic abilities in a negative form, they must look inside for the causal factor. If a psychic experiences attacking "demons", it is usually the experience of one's own negative elementals or thought forms. These can be released when seen visually by cancelling them, to transmute the energy. Truly, there is no evil, only ignorance. Even such things as can only occur if the person believes on a subconscious level that someone else can have power over him or her. Anyone who would try to possess another also does so out of ignorance, as cause will bring the effect back to them. For ages we have given much of our power away to the governments and religions. It is these institutions that really possess us. The blind following of governments or religions keeps the same emotional blocks and denial alive through each generation. We must break the chains of ignorance and mass hypnosis by removing the blocks that are located throughout our bodies, which were placed there as a result of the denial of who we truly are— co-creators with the universal life essence. Truly, we are beings of light, and the more we recognize this, the higher our collective vibration will become. It all evolves around true conscious awareness of who you are. Reiki can help this process by bringing back energy and balance to areas of the body which have been long denied the nurturing and healing qualities of the Life Force Energy. Devote some time to listen to your body, and feel the areas which may be blocked. Daily self-treatments, especially using the Second Degree mental healing technique, will help to release outmoded patterns of behaviour. You may experience long withheld emotions coming up, in addition to interesting dreams. As you get a sense of the cause of the block or denial, using your knowledge of the area of the body from which it comes, you can begin to formulate affirmation to permanently eradicate any negative thought forms. Using these tools and your own intuitive abilities, you will begin to formulate the appropriate program of healing and enlightenment.

# The Aura

In Latin, *Aura* means gently moving air, a breath of air, fragrance, light and a glow of light. The aura itself is an energy field which

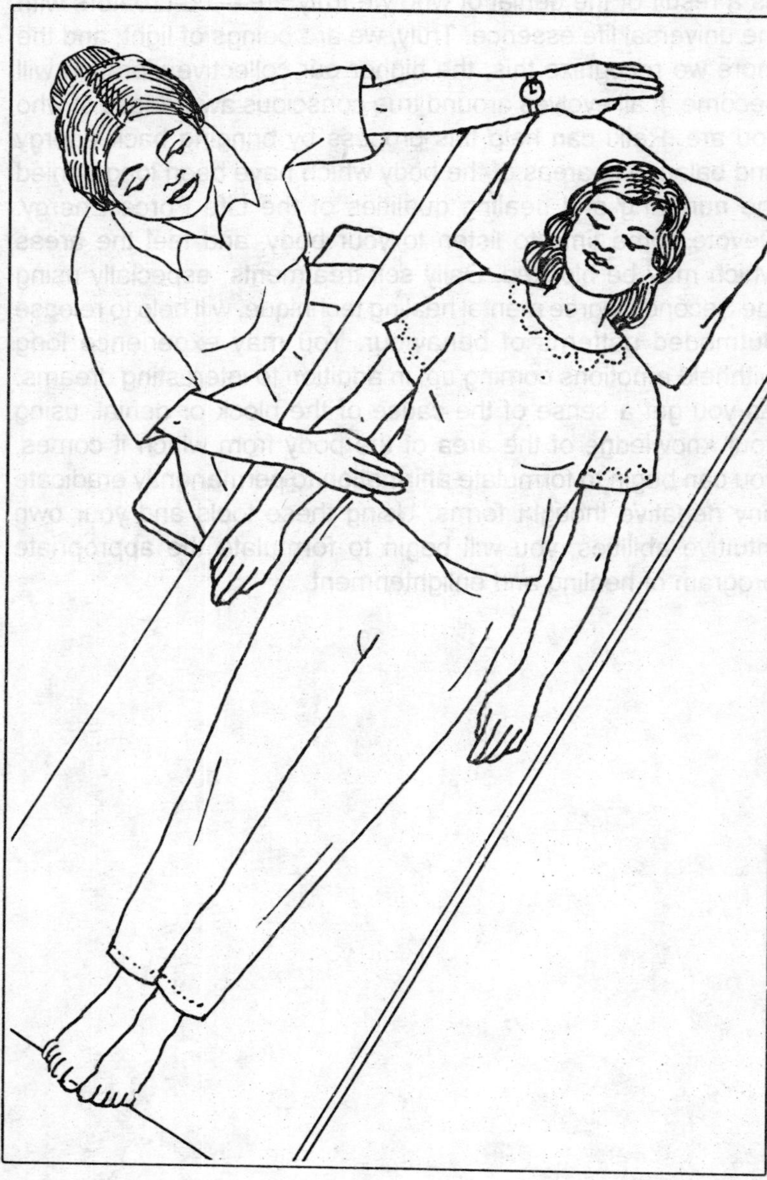

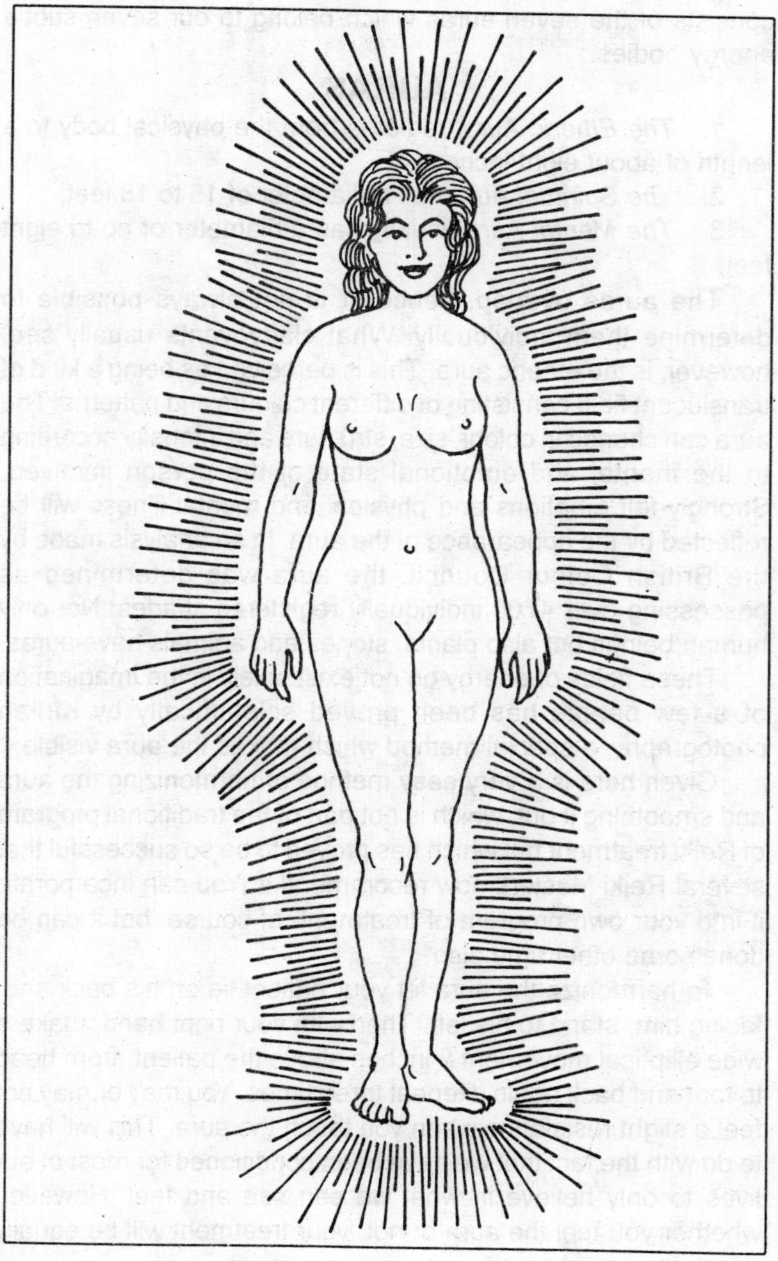

surrounds the body and permeates it, like a kind of halo. It consists of the seven auras which belong to our seven subtle energy bodies.

## AURAS

1. *The Etheric Aura,* radiates from the physical body to a length of about eight inches.

2. *The Spiritual Aura* has a diameter of 15 to 18 feet;

3. *The Mental Aura* usually has a diameter of up to eight feet.

The auras overlap, hence, it is not always possible to determine them individually. What clairvoyants usually see, however, is the etheric aura. This is perceived as being a kind of translucent field consisting of different colours and patterns. The aura can change in colour, size, structure and intensity according to the mental and emotional state of the person involved. Strongly-felt emotions and physical and mental illness will be reflected by the appearance of the aura. In an analysis made by the British Colour Council, the aura was determined as possessing over 4700 individually registered shades. Not only human beings but also plants, stones and animals have auras.

These fields of energy do not exist solely in the imagination of a few people has been proved scientifically by Kirlian photography, a special method which makes the aura visible.

Given here is a very easy method of harmonizing the aura and smoothing it out, which is not part of the traditional program of Reiki treatment but which has proved to be so successful that several Reiki Masters now recommend it. You can incorporate it into your own program of treatment, of course, but it can be done some other time also.

To harmonize the aura let your patient lie on his back and, facing him, stand to his left. Then with your right hand, make a wide elliptical movement 8 inches above the patient, from head to foot and back again. Repeat three times. You may or may not feel a slight resistance when you touch the aura. This will have to do with the fact that we have been conditioned for most of our lives to only believe in what we can see and feel. However, whether you feel the aura or not, your treatment will be equally effective and once you have started to look out for the aura, you will probably begin to feel it after some practice.

During Reiki session also you can make a try, when the patient is lying on his stomach. Here again, stand to the right of the patient and describe three ellipses in the air above his body, from head to foot and back again, that is all. This method will generally require no more than 12 seconds and will leave the patient feeling good as well as harmonizing him. Very sensitive people will sense their auras being smoothed out.

A method for loosening up the aura is also there, which can be done at any time but not as part of a Reiki session. It is very effective and helpful, especially when someone is depressed or weighed down. In this method the patient should stand in front of you with his eyes closed. Now, starting at the feet and working your way up, loosen up the aura as if you were whirling feathers into the air. Repeat from all sides, until the whole aura has been treated. This method will cheer people and help them feel lighter. Try it out and see the result.

# COMBINATION OF REIKI AND OTHER HEALING METHODS

According to modern age findings, Reiki will both support and increase the effectiveness of almost every kind of medication. Reiki blends well with a variety of different therapies, you already know about, which can be used in conjunction with Reiki treatments. One especially effective combination is used in conjunction with bodywork. Many massage therapists around the world combine Reiki treatment with Swedish, Circulatory, Sports, Acupressure, and Trigger Point massage, to name just a few. Other form of bodywork, such as Rolfing, Emotional Point Release Work, and Polarity, are enhanced with Reiki. The method for combining Reiki with body work is as under:

Start with the client lying face up. After doing a few minutes of neck massage, give a full scalp and deep facial massage. Next, perform all of the Reiki heal positions and continue to cover the entire endocrine/chakra system giving extra attention where needed. Complete Reiki on the front of the body by treating the knees and feet. Covering the knees is very important as they hold fear of death, fear of death of the old self or ego, and fear of change. All of us are going through intense changes these days, so a large amount of energy is needed in this area. Feet have points that connect with the entire body which makes them a nice place to finish Reiki on the front portion of the body. Now return to the shoulders and apply oil. Now it is time to begin the massage on the front of the body. Once the legs and feet are finished, the client is asked to turn over and oil is again applied to the back of the legs and the feet, and then the back itself. Once the massage is complete, Reiki is applied to the entire back, which is followed by a final energy balancing technique on the spine.

Only one suggestion for combining Reiki and massage is mentioned above. Using your intuition as a guide, the possibilities for combining the various techniques are many.

Combination of Reiki and allopathic medicine is also very effective. Doctors can use Reiki to feel where the energy is being drawn, while at the same time, actually transmitting healing energy to their patients. It can also be used in the process of setting bones to diminish pain, and accelerate the healing process. Even pediatricians can use it in the care and handling of young children. More and more doctors are becoming interested in Reiki as they discover the myriad of ways that it can be used to enhance their treatments. Reiki also can help to improve the effectiveness of medication. Through the wonderful work of Dolores Krienger and Therapeutic Touch, the benefits of hands on healing have gained great acceptance in the medical field. With the amplified energy of Reiki, hands-on healing takes on a new dimension. Many nurses are being drawn to Reiki as they search for alternative healing methods which provide more personal contact, as well as a regenerative tool to use with their patients. Infants, as well as, children and adults in intensive care units, benefit greatly from the treatments. Patients are comforted by the energy provided by Reiki.

Ayurvedic, Naturopathic and Homeopathic treatments are also enhanced with Reiki. Charging remedies with Reiki is a powerful tool for accelerating healing energy. Another powerful healing method used in combination with Reiki is fasting.

Fasting is one of the oldest methods used since ages to cure complications like arthritis, asthma, skin problems, high blood pressure, digestive disorders, and kidney and liver diseases. Most diseases in man are self-induced through overeating, poor diet, and lack of exercise. Lethargy and overindulging in rich foods is a sure path to autointoxication. Disease then results when glandular activity and metabolic rate slow down, and the eliminative organs decrease in efficiency due to the steady build-up of toxic deposits in the cells and tissues of the body. For example, rheumatoid arthritis is a result of uric acid crystals and mineral compounds which have collected in the joints and soft tissues. High blood pressure, along with stress, is a result of metabolic wastes which have been deposited in the arteries and small blood capillaries, resulting in a restriction in the blood flow. Fasting is a very powerful method for expelling all the waste products from our system.

After two days of fasting autolysis begins to occur. After 72 hours without food, the body starts to digest its own waste materials. The first to be digested are always unnecessary toxins which are stored in the body, such as cysts, tumours, and excess mineral build-ups. These are followed by the digestion of excess fatty tissue. It is also after the third day that the initial discomforts of feeling hungry, and possible dizziness or weakness all disappear. In Scandinavia, doctors who follow the biological route for curing their patients, use fasts anywhere from seven to sixty days in duration, with truly amazing results. If a patient is very weak or sick to begin with, they will be put on a healthy diet to build up strength, and later, ask them to start fasting.

There are many different fasts. Some are pure water fasts, and others combine fruit juices and vegetable both. The key to any fast is to use only fresh fruits and vegetables. Using a juicer to make the appropriate drink just before you imbibe it is the ideal, in order to benefit from the raw live enzymes. One of the most popular cancer cures developed in the 20's and 30's, initially to cure tuberculosis, and later cancer, in the Max Gerson therapy, which is based on the premise that raw live foods act to cleanse and naturally strengthen the immune system of the body.

During fasting, it is important to not only drink plenty of liquid, but it is also important to give yourself a couple of enemas each day to make sure that the bowels are kept clear of toxic materials. After three days of fasting, there is not always enough falcal matter to sustain parastaltic action, however, the toxins do still build up in the intestines, thus it is important to keep yourself flushed out to avoid autotoxicity. For those who are interested in fasting, it is suggested that you consult a wholistically oriented physician if you are trying it for the first time, because he may be able to tell you about the detailed plan and the appropriate way to come off a fast.

Reiki is of great use with fasting, it will help to alleviate any of the symptoms which might occur in the first three days. Also, it amplifies the Life Force Energy in the body, which helps to boost the immune system, and speed up the process of elimination. For those pursuing a wholistic oriented biological cure, fasting, used in combination with Reiki, will produce desired results for them.

Though fasting provides a very effective means for cleansing the physical body and eliminating years of toxic build-up, but there may be times in life when we seek to clear out old and inappropriate negative emotional patterns, in order to create a more positive approach to life. The healing of the emotional body is just as important as healing the physical body. As stress and tension become stored in the body, and begin to mould its form over the years, the personality becomes moulded as well. We tend to develop negative reactive habit patterns when we subject ourselves to constant emotional stress. To help release these patterns, which extend all the way back to the birth trauma, a technique called Rebirthing or "Conscious Breathing" has been used for over fifteen years. The original founder, Leonard Orr, began the development of Rebirthing in the early 1970's. Many sessions are completed in jacuzzis heated to body temperature, in order to effect a womb-like environment. A relaxed rhythmic breathing is employed with each inhalation and exhalation, connected in one long unbroken chain. The breath is focused in the lungs or chest, rather than the diaphragm, and it is appropriate to breathe out of either the nose or mouth. The primary goal of the breathing is to move energy through the body. During the rebirthing process, it is common to feel tingling and vibrating sensations throughout the entire body. Many people experience a stiffening of the hands due to the release of long accumulated tensions, and resistance to the energy flowing throughout the body. This is usually a signpost that a great deal of sadness is coming up and needs to be released. These symptoms come and go very quickly as the breathing pattern is continued. As each thought form is turned from negative to positive, with the help of rebirther, much healing takes place. It is recommended that several sessions are carried out until you experience what Orr calls the Breath Release. This occurs when you re-experience your first breath. It evokes a powerful healing as the damage done at birth to the breathing pattern is healed, and your habit of improper breathing vanishes.

There is another development in conscious breathing that is the tendency in some people to regress back to past life memories. What is important to note is that whether we have lived before or not, these memories of past lives do exist. There are a variety of explanations, however, what is important is that these "stories" act as powerful tools to help one release long buried emotions and shed light on our sometimes inappropriate reactions to certain situations at present.

Most of the problems in this life are connected with images and sensations from past lives. When you re-experience these memories fully, the problems in this life begin to disappear. For example, if you have problems in relationship, you will most likely see and experience scenes and images during a regression utilizing conscious breathing, that are connected to those same relationship problems. You are then able to let them go and transform them. You also will begin to perceive your problems in a different light, as you start to understand your present behavioural patterns, as they relate to past life situations.

Experiences with rebirthing may prove to be very beneficial, because they enable a person to release long and deeply buried emotions, while freeing up his psyche to new and more positive ways of being in the world.

Rebirthing is an important healing tool, and when used in combination with Reiki, many positive changes can occur.

Anyone with the willingness to allow growth and change in the life, will find Reiki and Rebirthing to be a very effective combination.

There are various other therapies which may be used together with Reiki. Use it in your area of expertise, and allow its supportive energies to assist you in the creation of your own healing form. But remember, Reiki is not a substitute for every kind of medication and treatment, but it will help in biological healing process.

# GROUP OR TEAM TREATMENT

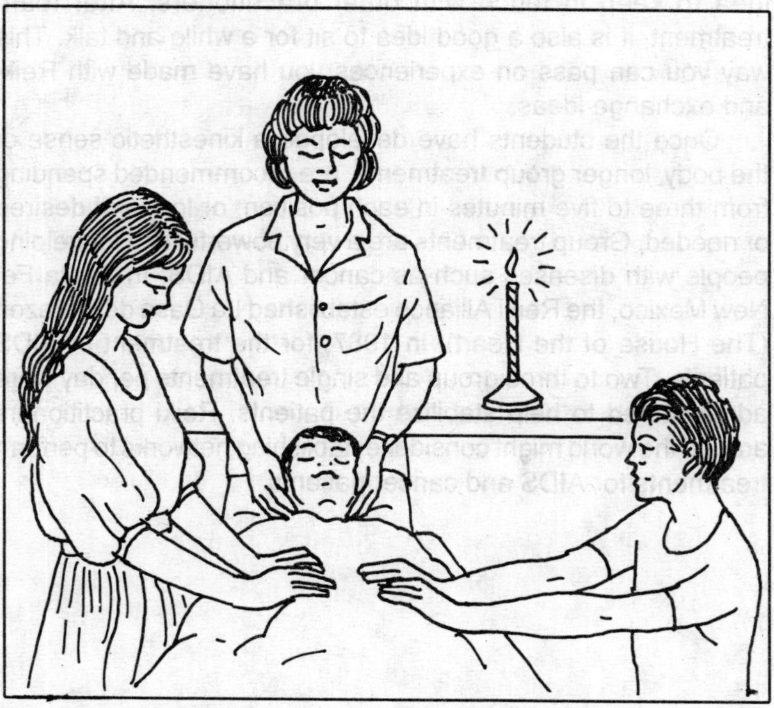

In such conditions when more than one person treats at the same time, there is extraordinary increase in healing energy. Group treatments are a wonderful way to share the Reiki energy among friends. Group treatments are usually shorter than formal one-on-one treatments, as the full body is covered by several people. The energy is also amplified as a result of so many channels treating a patient.

You will feel fine if you would treat someone with Reiki with other practitioners at the same time. This method not only increases the effectiveness of treatment, it is also shorter while being a lot more enjoyable.

Dr. Hayashi, the former Grand Master, let his patient be treated by several practitioners at once in his Reiki clinic in Tokyo, Japan. Before starting treatment, it is important to decide who should start off and which sequence should be followed, but this is not something to discuss in front of the patient. Treating with several practitioners at once has proved especially valuable in difficult and stubborn cases and, for this reason, it is a good idea to keep in touch with other practitioners. After team treatment, it is also a good idea to sit for a while and talk. This way you can pass on experiences you have made with Reiki and exchange ideas.

Once the students have developed a kinesthetic sense of the body, longer group treatments, are recommended spending from three to five minutes in each position, or longer if desired or needed. Group treatments are a very powerful tool for helping people with diseases such as cancer and AIDS. In Santa Fe, New Mexico, the Reiki Alliance established La Casa de Corazon (The House of the Heart), in 1987, for the treatment of AIDS patients. Two to three group and single treatments per day were administered to help stabilize the patients. Reiki practitioners around the world might consider establishing networks to perform treatments for AIDS and cancer patients.

# THE MENTAL HEALING

Negative experiences change our attitude towards life and behaviour. This kind of unconscious programming makes us attract the same distressful experiences over and over again, almost in confirmation of our worst hopes. It is often very difficult to free ourselves of such ingrained patterns of behaviour, even when we know the causes. Here the mental healing method, which is taught in Second Degree Reiki, can be of great help. (The word "mental" is derived from the Latin *mens,* which has the meaning of "to think," "the thinker," "consciousness" and "concerning the spirit." *Mens* also corresponds to the Sanskrit word *manas* from which the word "man" is derived.)

By using the right kind of "key," it is possible to come into contact with the innermost being of a person and to change his inner "program" in such a way that his misdirected energy will be transformed and set free. In this way, depression can be changed into the joy of life, and fear will become trust. Lack of courage will turn into optimism and an inferiority complex can be transformed into inner wealth. Hate will become love and happiness, and a positive attitude will arise out of negative one.

More often the patient will gain insight into his behaviour and recognize the cause of his problems with the help of the mental method. Moreover, it will also help him recognize and achieve his goal quite easily.

Physical illness is usually a manifestation of spiritual imbalance, hence, the mental healing method can be used in the case of all psychic disturbances. In order to help you identify programs which often occur with certain kinds of ailments.

Just like self-treatment and absentee healing, the mental technique is usually given as part of a normal Reiki treatment, but it only lasts a few minutes. However, this form of treatment requires a great sense of responsibility on the part of the practitioner. A lot of thought should go into giving it, and it should only be carried out with the patient's permission. The practitioner should not thrust his own ideas and value judgements onto his patient. Instead, his sole consideration should be his well-being.

The mental method can also be applied to plants and animals and is a truly wonderful and beneficial instrument with which you will be able to achieve many desired goals.

Not only should there be an exchange of energy for treatments, but there should also be an exchange of energy for Reiki classes. Teachers seek students who are ready to receive the Reiki energy and are willing to earn it. It is important that a student appreciates and is prepared for the benefits of Reiki. The underlying principle is the same as that which Dr. Usui discovered after his years in the Beggars Quarter. He had seen many people come and go, and had also seen many return to their old ways. He decided to seek out people who really wanted to transform themselves. One should not waste precious time and energy sharing information or energy with those who are not interested or prepared to receive or do not feel gratitude.

How does one become a professional Reiki practitioner? The answer is different in each country. In Physicians, Nurses, Massage Therapists, Physiotherapists, Chiropractors, Acupuncture Doctors, Naturopaths, Homeopaths, and Ayurvedic Doctors all have license to touch the body and can readily blend Reiki with their treatments. Many psychologists are also adding Reiki to their practices, due to the powerful emotional healing technique introduced in Second Degree. A specific fee cannot be charged, but you can suggest a donation. In Germany, such a process is unfortunately not available. You can use cards advertising Reiki as a Relaxation Technique, as long as you do not use the word therapy. It is your responsibility to find out the specific laws that affect the area in which you live.

There should always be fair exchange of energy. This can be money or the natural give-and-take. Dr Usui had said, "I cut off all beggers. Never again Reiki be given away. Always there will have to an exchange with Reiki". As far as an exchange of energy is concerned, the fee for a Reiki treatment should be considered comparable to the fee for an hour of massage therapy in your area.But remember, you should never make a diagnosis unless you are a doctor. If you strongly sense that something is very wrong, you may refer a person to a qualified doctor for a proper diagnosis. Also, never prescribe drugs or suggest that someone discontinue them.

One key piece of advice is that a person who needs Reiki treatment must ask for that, you must not also feel obligated to oblige if you are not too inclined. It is very important to realize that sometimes people derive secondary benefits from illness. Although they may ask for a healing on a conscious level, they may not really want to be healed. For example, someone who frequently lacks attention from a mate or a parent, may find that all the attention that he or she receives while ill is a difficult thing to give up. If you treat someone for a while, and your intuition begins to tell you that they are becoming overly dependent on you, and that they need to take full responsibility for their own healing, you should take steps to release them. One simple way to break this gently to a client is to tell them that your inner guidance has advised you that they are quite capable of healing themselves, and that there is nothing more that you can do for them at this time. You might suggest that they take a Reiki class and learn to treat themselves, or give them a creative visualization or affirmation that they can use. It is really important to know when it is time to release a client, the purpose of this practice is to promote responsible, consciously aware individuals.If you are dependent on the income earned this way, then it is recommended that you let the patient pay whatever he feels fit or accept payment in the form of a donation.

Making an exchange of energy is an important part of the healing process. It saves people from the burden of obligation, and also it helps them to have an investment in the end result. The exchange should be in proportion to the person's income, and does not necessarily need to involve money. The give and take of Reiki, is truly one of its important assets. To live in a balanced, harmonious world, we must be comfortable with both giving and receiving.This is what exchange of energy is all about. Many people have difficulty charging for Reiki treatments. But they should always remember that they are charging for their time.

# REIKI CIRCLE

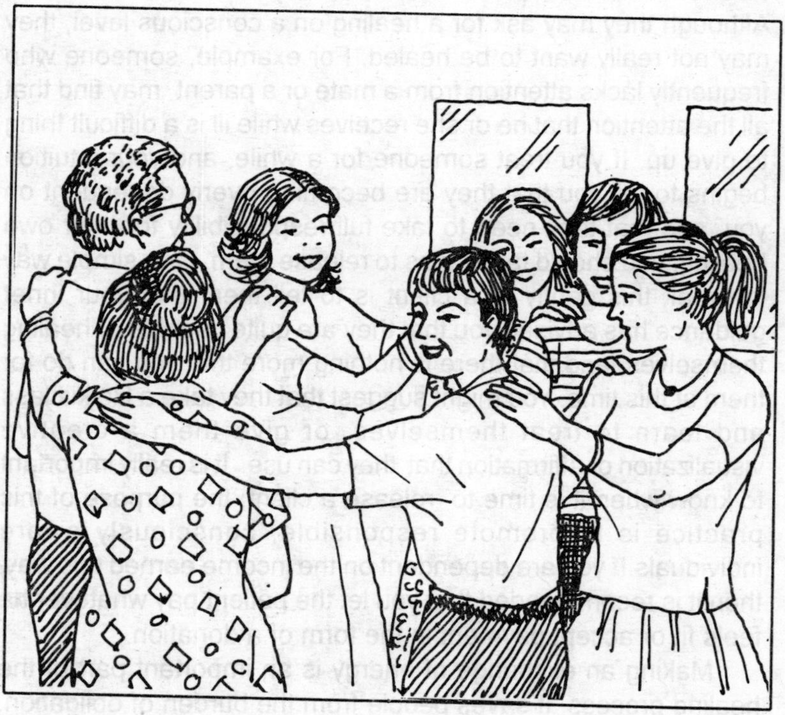

When you take part in a large meeting of Reiki practitioners, you will be able to fill the ancient symbol of the circle with new life again. The circle stands for infinity and perfection and by forming one, you can create a never-ending-ever-beginning circle of Reiki. To do this, sit or stand in a circle and lay your hands on the shoulders or waist of the person to your left. Now start to let Reiki flow. The effect will be more pleasant if the group is quiet and united. This is a very beautiful and effective way of activating and putting Reiki energy to use within a whole group. This wonderful experience of giving and receiving will promote the feeling of unity within a group and increase its harmony. With time, more and more people will start to rediscover the ancient symbols of old, and awaken them to new life.

If a lot of practitioners are present, the circle can be extended into a *spiral,* combining the energy of Reiki with the power contained in this *symbol.*

To know more sbout Spiral and Symbol read *The Mystical Spiral* by Jill Purse and *Man and His Symbols* by C.G. Jung.

# ENERGY EXCHANGE

After spending many years in the Beggars Quarter of Kyoto, Dr. Usui learned first hand about the importance of an exchange of energy for the healer's time. When he first became empowered to perform the miracle healings he had sought for so long, his initial thought was to move to the Beggars Quarter in true Christian style and serve the poor. His intention was to help heal them so that they could become responsible citizens, and enable them to hold a job to support themselves. What he discovered over time was that many returned after having experienced a taste of life on the outside, and decided that they didn't want the responsibility of caring for themselves. By just giving away healings, he had further impressed the beggar pattern in many of them. People needed to give back for what they received in order to fully appreciate what had been given.

Usui thus discovered two very important factors: One, that a person should ask for a healing (It is not the job of any healer to try and help where healing is not wanted): and two, that there should be an exchange of energy for the healer's time (It is not right to keep someone feeling indebted for services rendered. Thus the healee, by sharing energy in a variety of forms, frees himself of obligation).

This exchange of energy does not necessarily have to be in the form of money. It can be in the form of a trade of some sort. If the person requesting one or more treatments is a family member or very close friend, there is normally an exchange of energy taking place all of the time, so there need not be a request for specific reimbursement.

Not only should there be an exchange of energy for treatments, but there should also be an exchange of energy for Reiki classes. Teachers seek students who are ready to receive the Reiki energy and are willing to earn it. It is important that a student appreciates and is prepared for the benefits of Reiki. The underlying principle is the same as that which Dr. Usui discovered after his years in the Beggars Quarter. He had seen many people come and go, and had also seen many return to their old ways. Usui decided to seek out people who really wanted to transform themselves. One should not waste precious time and energy sharing information or energy with those who are not interested or prepared to receiver or do not feel gratitude.

How does one become a professional Reiki practitioner? The answer is different in each country. In many countries, Physicians, Nurses, Massage Therapists, Physiotherapists, Chiropractors, Acupuncture Doctors, Naturopaths, Homeopaths, and Ayurvedic Doctors all have license to touch the body and can readily blend Reiki with their treatments. Many psychologists are also adding Reiki to their practices, due to the powerful emotional healing technique introduced in Second Degree. A specific fee cannot be charged, but you can suggest a donation. In Germany, such a process is unfortunately not available. You can use cards advertising Reiki as a Relaxation Technique, as long as you do not use the word therapy. It is your responsibility to find out the specific laws that affect the area in which you live.

There should always be fair exchange of energy. This can be money or the natural give-and-take Dr Usui had said, "I cut off all beggers. Never again Reiki be given away. Always there will have to be an exchange with Reiki". As far as an exchange of energy is concerned, the fee for a Reiki treatment should be considered comparable to the fee for an hour of massage therapy in your area. But remember, you should never make a diagnosis unless you are a doctor. If you strongly sense that something is very wrong, you may refer a person to a qualified doctor for a proper diagnosis. Also, never prescribe drugs or suggest that someone discontinue them.

One key piece of advice is that a person who needs Reiki treatment must ask for that, you must not also feel obligated to oblige if you are not so inclined. It is very important to realize that sometimes people derive secondary benefits from illness. Although they may ask for a healing on a conscious level, they may not really want to be healed. For example, someone who frequently lacks attention from a mate or a parent, may find that all the attention that he or she receives while ill is a difficult thing to give up. If you treat someone for awhile, and your intuition begins to tell you that they are becoming overly dependent on you, and that they need to take full responsibility for their own healing, you should take steps to release them. One simple way to break this gently to a client is to tell them that your inner guidance has advised you that they are quite capable of healing themselves, and that there is nothing more that you can do for them at this time. You might suggest that they take a Reiki class and learn to treat themselves, or give them a creative visualization or affirmation that they can use. It is really important to know when it is time to release a client. The purpose of this practice is to promote responsible, consciously aware individuals.

If you are dependent on the income earned this way, then it is recommended that you let the patient pay whatever he feels fit or accept payment in the form of donation.

Making an exchange of energy is an important part of the healing process. It saves people from the burden of obligation, and also it helps them to have an investment in the end result. The exchange should be in proportion to the person's income, and does not necessarily need to involve money. The give and take of Reiki, is truly one of its important assets. To live in a balanced, harmonious world, we must be comfortable with both giving and receiving. This is what exchange of energy is all about. Many people have difficulty charging for Reiki treatments. But they should always remember that they are not charging for healing. Reiki does the healing-they are just charging for their time.

Where's the use of sighing?
Sorrow as you may,
Time is always flying —
Flying! — and defying
Men to say him way.

# REIKI FOR INFANTS, ANIMALS, FOOD AND ASSORTED ODDS AND ENDS

Reiki treatments are good for pregnant woman, because they help to alleviate some of the minor and major complaints of pregnancy, such as morning sickness in the first trimester, and later, lower back pain. Reiki also helps to soothe women as the emotions begin to fluctuate due to the large amount of hormones being released in the system. A mother often holds her baby lovingly anyway and once she has learned to give Reiki she can pass it on to her baby each time she strokes and touches it. This higher form of energy will intensify the natural relationship between mother and child and make it finer. Moreover, everything the infant human being experiences in its first weeks, months and years condition it for life. Whoever received a lot of love and affection as a baby will generally be able to pass on these qualities himself when he becomes older.

The people who know Reiki and like gardening are well aware of the benefits that plants derive from being treated. Seeds that are treated before being planted, tend to grow into healthier plants than those which are not treated. Hold them between the palms of your hands and treat them as long as they draw energy. Seed sprouts in the earth can be treated by holding your hands just above them. Regular treatments given to your vegetable garden helps to produce an abundance of vital healthy plants. Flowers and shrubs do very well too when treated with Reiki. Blossoms tend to proliferate, and the growth of shrubs is accelerated. Cut flowers tend to last longer when supported with Reiki, and indoor plants also react in miraculous ways. Potted plants are best treated via roots, with the pot held between hands as a flower-vase.

Trees can be given Reiki too. They take it through their trunk, hence you should hug them to treat them with Reiki.

Much has been written about the secret life of plants. Scientific tests have been done to show how plants react to our emotions, and to music. It has also been found that talking to plants helps to aid in the development of a healthy specimen.

Although we don't know what animals experience when they receive Reiki, but it can be clearly noticed that they tend to get quieter and relaxed. Occasionally you will find a rare animal who rejects the energy, and that must be respected. The average animal, however, will experience the same benefits that humans do. The fact that animals are healed with Reiki treatment tends to prove that the belief system has little effect on the outcome of the Reiki healing.

The anatomy of animal is very similar to human anatomy, so, when treating a specific organ in an animal's body, you can judge its position fairly easily by its placement in your own body. Also, as with treating humans, special attention should be given to areas which draw larger amounts of energy. Covering the endocrine system, when possible, is also recommended.

In such conditions when an animal is very restless, or it seems dangerous to treat with hands-on treatment, absentee healings can be utilized. Patting an animal before treatment is one way to soothe it. You can then follow your intuition in the placement of your hands.

Reiki can also be put to a variety of other uses. We must keep in mind that all matter is vibration at different levels of density— that everything on the physical plane is composed of universal life force energy in different phases of evolution. As all matter is vibration, Reiki can penetrate anything, much like the etheric substance of your body which permeates your environment. It is also possible to clear an environment such as a room with Reiki energy, to remove any negative etheric substance. Reiki is generally used for situations where there is a deficiency or lack of harmony, it can also be used to enrich things with additional life energy, such as food, medicine, plasters, bandages, clothes and shoes, as well as pieces of jewellery and gems.

Some people will be surprised to learn that cars can also be treated. These objects actually tend to take on the etheric energy of their owners and become affected by our moods. If your car won't start in winter, try treating it with Reiki first, putting your hands around the battery for a few minutes before starting up the engine again. They become the anima to our animus or the animus to our anima. When the two are not in harmony, Reiki treatments are called for, because they can help you to avoid undesirable breakdowns and mechanical mishaps. With a little thought, you will find many more ways of putting Reiki to use in everyday life. The food can be enhanced by treating it with Reiki. In most countries around the world, people tend to eat an excessive amount of cooked or "dead" foods. The raw foods provide live enzymes which keep the body young and healthy and prevent the deterioration which causes quick aging in most of the human race. A raw food diet is an important factor in health. When you are in situations which prevent you from obtaining the correct amount of raw life foods, you can enhance your cooked food with the universal life force energy of Reiki. After treating and having your food, you may also treat your belly to accelerate digestion process.

All matter is composed of the Universal Life Force Energy at different levels of vibration. Reiki, which is a channeled and intensified form of this energy, can be used to energize not only living breathing life forms, but also "solid" matter. Try Reiki wherever you can and see the difference.

# BODY PSYCHOLOGY AND EMOTION CENTERS

It is important to know that where emotions are stored in body. The brain is an organ which registers and retains thoughts and memories. However, the mind itself actually functions through the etheric body and leaves its impressions throughout the entire physical structure. The matter that we take into our bodies helps to shape our physical structures, and by the same token, the thoughts we project, and the emotional reactions that pass through our bodies, also affects its form and texture. Thus the body is a reflection of the mind, and in turn, as the body develops in certain ways, the mind will act as a reflection of the body. The body's tissues will actually adjust their size and texture according to the quality of emotions and thoughts passing through it. Positive energy will help to keep the body flexible and supple, whereas suppressed actions of desires will tend to create energy blocks in the etheric and then physical bodies. Blocked energy will actually form rigidity in the tissue. Different parts of body take up different function as follows :

***Abdomen***

- contains deepest feelings
- center of sexuality
- digestive system
- center of emotions

***Abductors***

- inner thigh
- contain sexually charged tissues

***Ankles***

- create balance

***Arm (upper)***

- strength to act
- fear of being discouraged

***Arms***

- enable us to move
- connect in the external world
- express the heart center, love

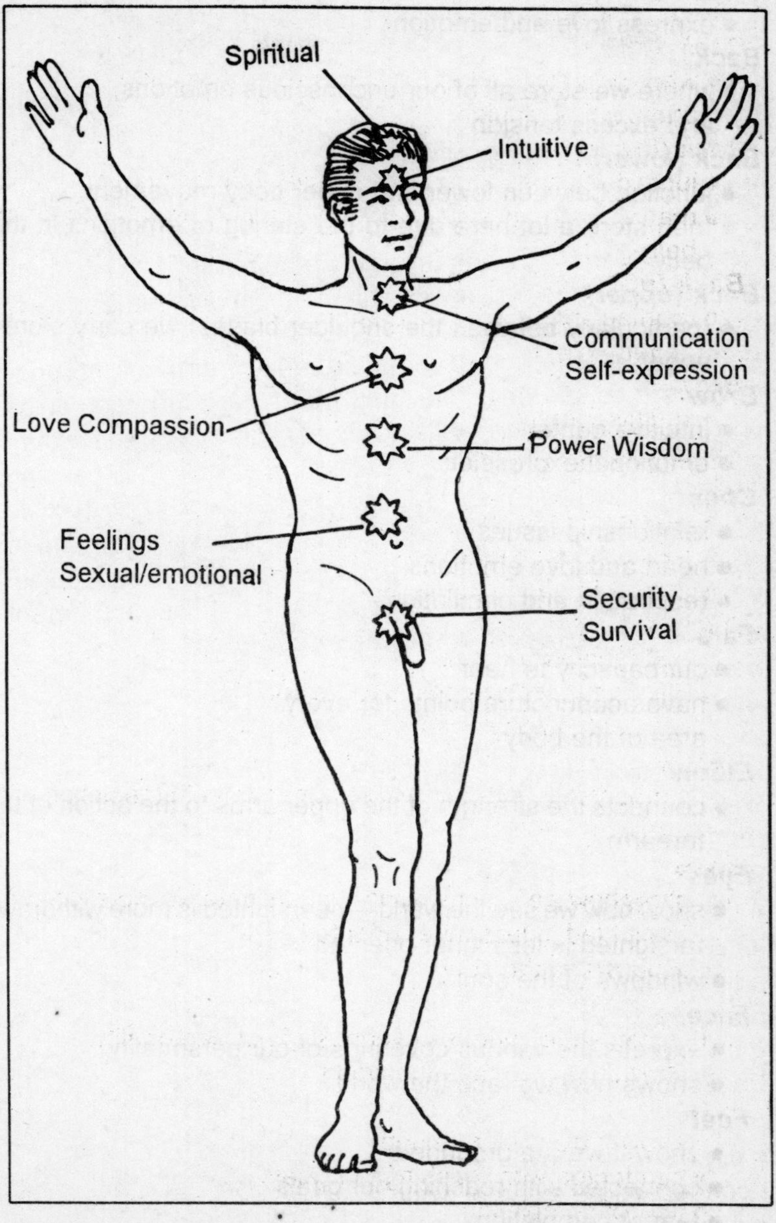
Spiritual
Intuitive
Communication
Self-expression
Love Compassion
Power Wisdom
Feelings
Sexual/emotional
Security
Survival

***Arms and hands***

- are extensions of the heart center
- express love and emotion

***Back***

- where we store all of our unconscious emotions, and excess tension

***Back (lower)***

- junction between lower and upper body movement
- men store a lot here due to the storing of emotions in the belly

***Back (upper)***

- (particularly between the shoulder blades) we carry stored anger

***Brow***

- intuitive center
- emotional expression

***Chest***

- relationship issues
- heart and love emotions
- respiration and circulation

***Ears***

- our capacity to hear
- have acupuncture points for every area of the body

***Elbow***

- connects the strength of the upper arms to the action of the forearm

***Eyes***

- show how we see the world— nearsighted is more withdrawn farsighted is less inner oriented
- windows of the soul

***Face***

- express the various coverings of our personality
- shows how we face the world

***Feet***

- show if we are grounded
- connected with reaching our goals
- fear of completion

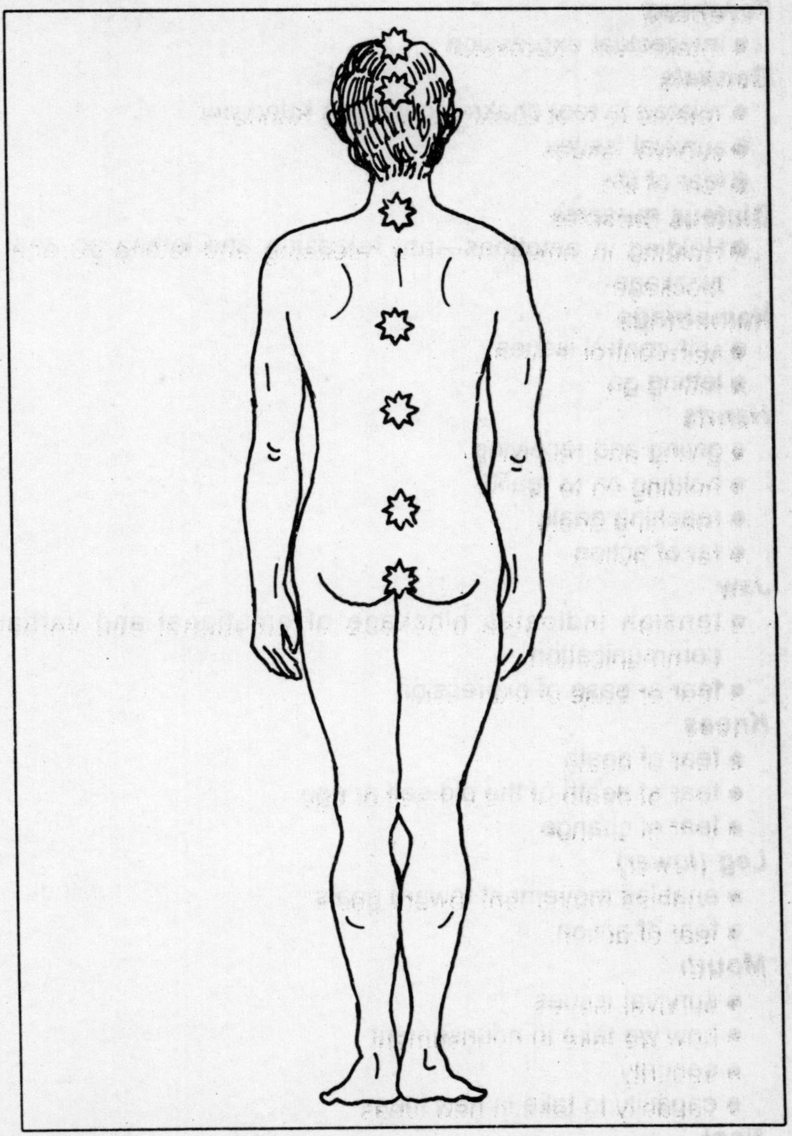

***Forearm***

- means of attaining goals
- fear of inferiority

***Forehead***

- intellectual expression

***Genitals***

- related to root chakra containing Kundalini
- survival issues
- fear of life

***Gluteus muscles***

- Holding in emotions—not releasing and letting go anal blockage

***Hamstrings***

- self-control issues
- letting go

***Hands***

- giving and receiving
- holding on to reality
- reaching goals
- far of action

***Jaw***

- tension indicates blockage of emotional and verbal communication
- fear or ease of expression

***Knees***

- fear of death
- fear of death of the old-self or ego
- fear of change

***Leg (lower)***

- enables movement toward goals
- fear of action

***Mouth***

- survival issues
- how we take in nourishment
- security
- capacity to take in new ideas

***Neck***

- thought and emotions come
- together

- stiffness is due to withheld
- statements

***Nose***

- related to heart (colouration and bulbousness)
- sense and smell, sexual response self-recognition

***Pelvis***

- seat of Kundalini energy
- root of basic survival needs and actions

***Shoulders***

- where we carry the weight of the world
- fear of responsibility
- women store a lot here

***Solar Plexus***

- power issues
- emotional control issues
- power wisdom center

***Thigh***

- personal strength
- trust in one's own abilities
- fear of inadequate strength

## Division of front and back

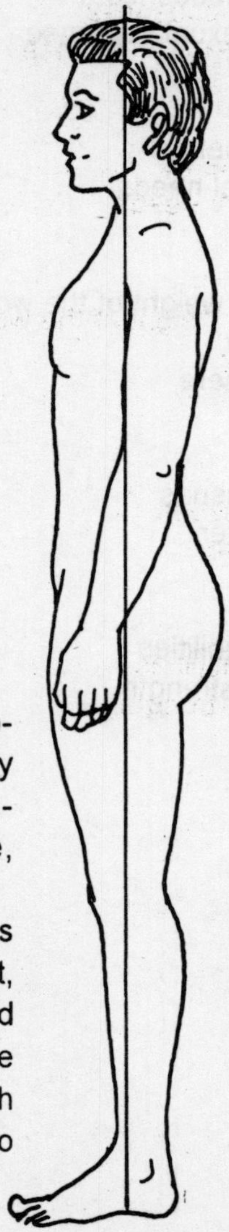

***Front :*** A mirror
- — Social mask
- — contains the emotional issues of daily life, such as: concern, love, desire, sadness, joy, etc.
- — heartfelt pain is stored in the chest, between the ribs and the insides of the shoulders. Much emotion is also stored in the belly

***Back :*** many of our unconscious thoughts and emotions are stored here
- — here we hide issues we are not prepared to handle
- — it is our emotional disposal area for all the things we don't want to acknowledge
- — plenty of fear and anger is stored between the shoulder blades, and along the spinalis muscle on either side of the spine

## Division of right and left sides

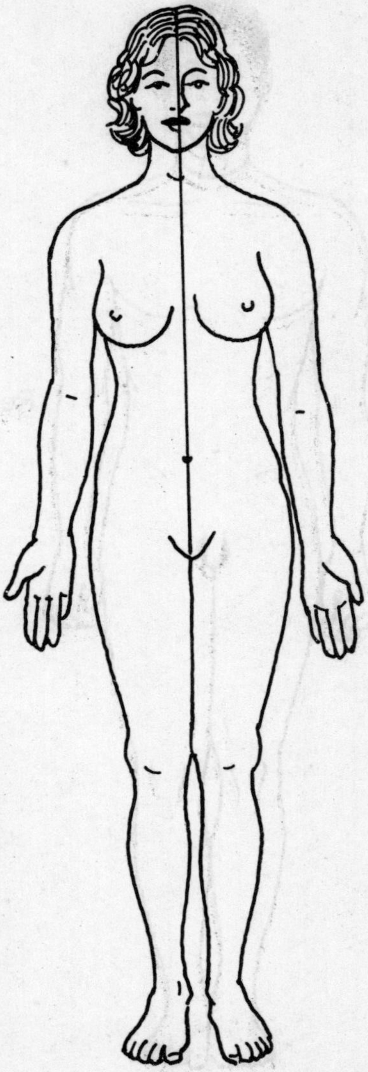

*Right side :*
Masculine
— assertive
— yang
— male aspects of character
— holds anger
— logical, rational

*Left side*
Ferminine
— receptive
— passive
— yin
— feminine aspects of character
—holds sadness
— intuitive

## Division of Head/Body

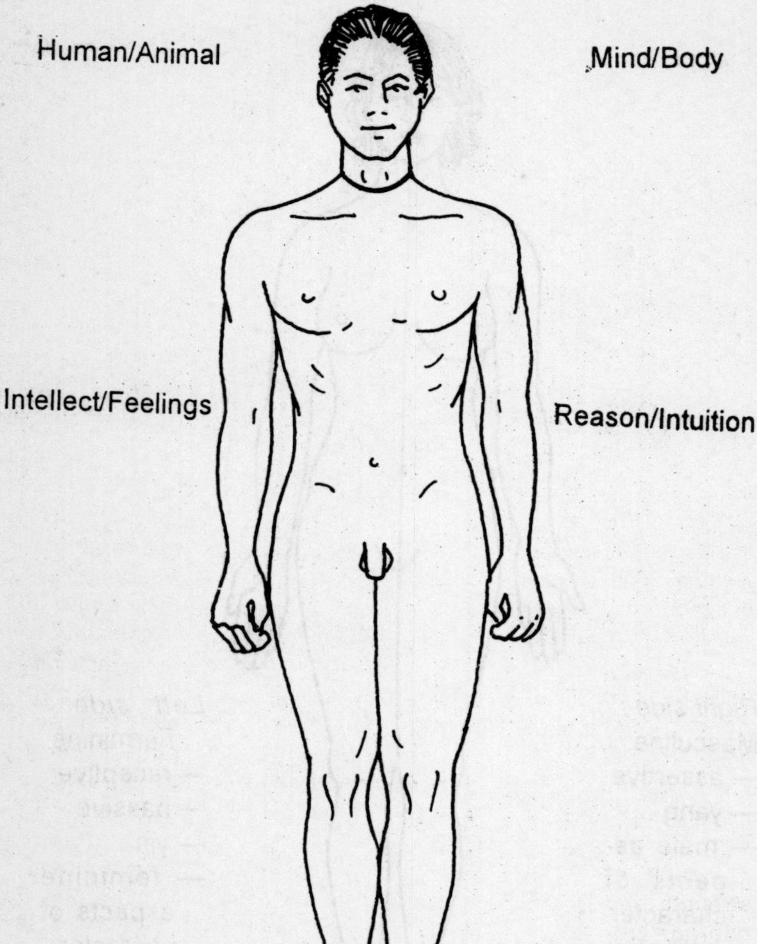

## Division of Top/Bottom

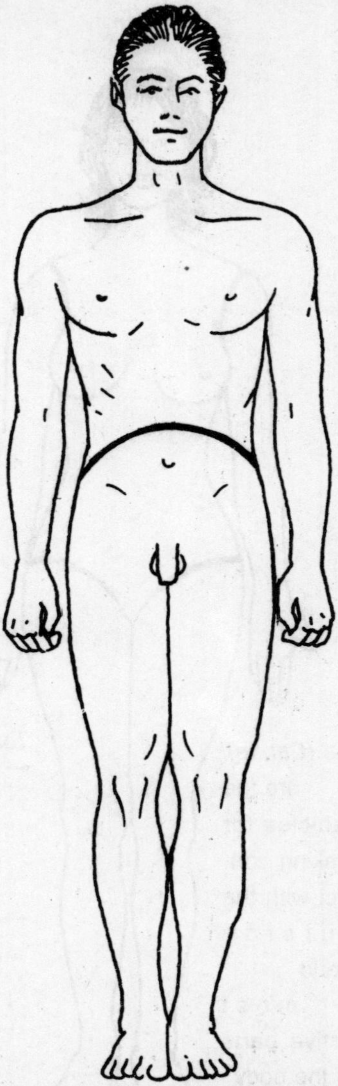

*Large Top/Small Bottom*
(mostly found in males)
— overdeveloped in ability to be assertive, social expressive, extroverted
— lack of strength and courage regarding emotional stability and support
— active personality

*Small Top/Large Bottom*
(mostly found in females)
— finds difficulty in outward expression, interpersonal communications, socializing self-assertion, and taking action
— prefer privacy, home well grounded, stable.
— passive personality

## Division or Limb and Torso

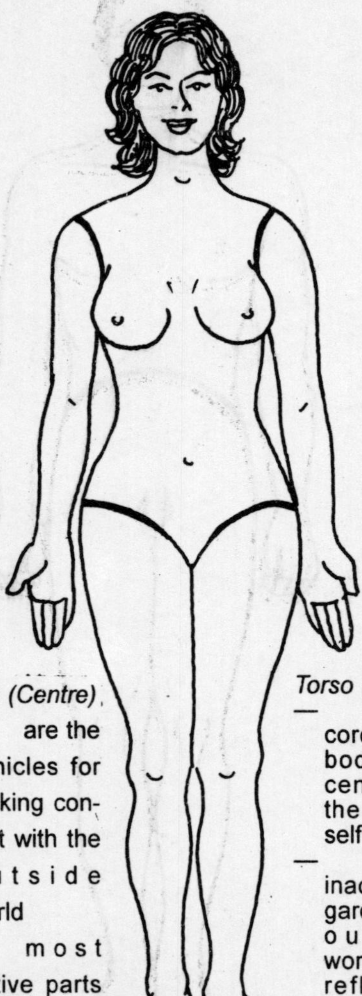

*Limbs (Centre)*

— are the vehicles for making contact with the outside world

— most active parts of the body

*Torso (Centre)*

— is the core of the body, the center of the private self

— very inactive regarding the outside world more reflective, focused on the self

## The Emotional Release Points in the Frontside

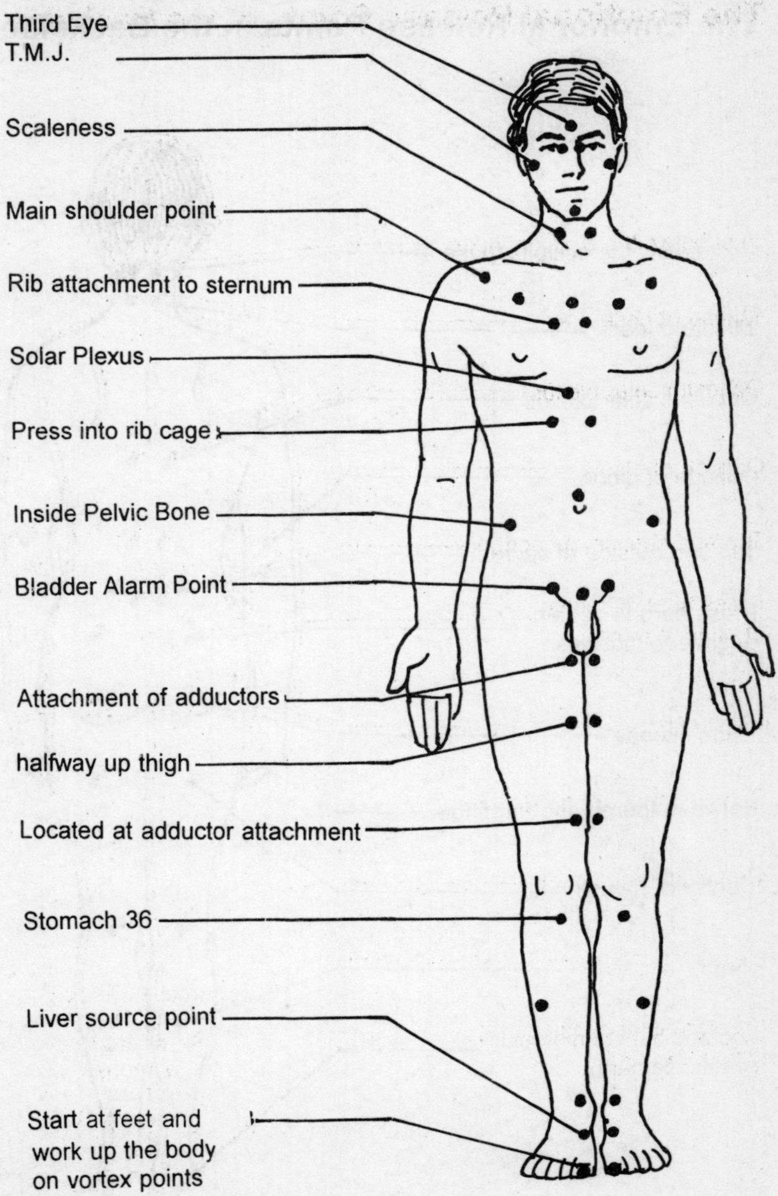

# The Emotional Release Points in the Backside

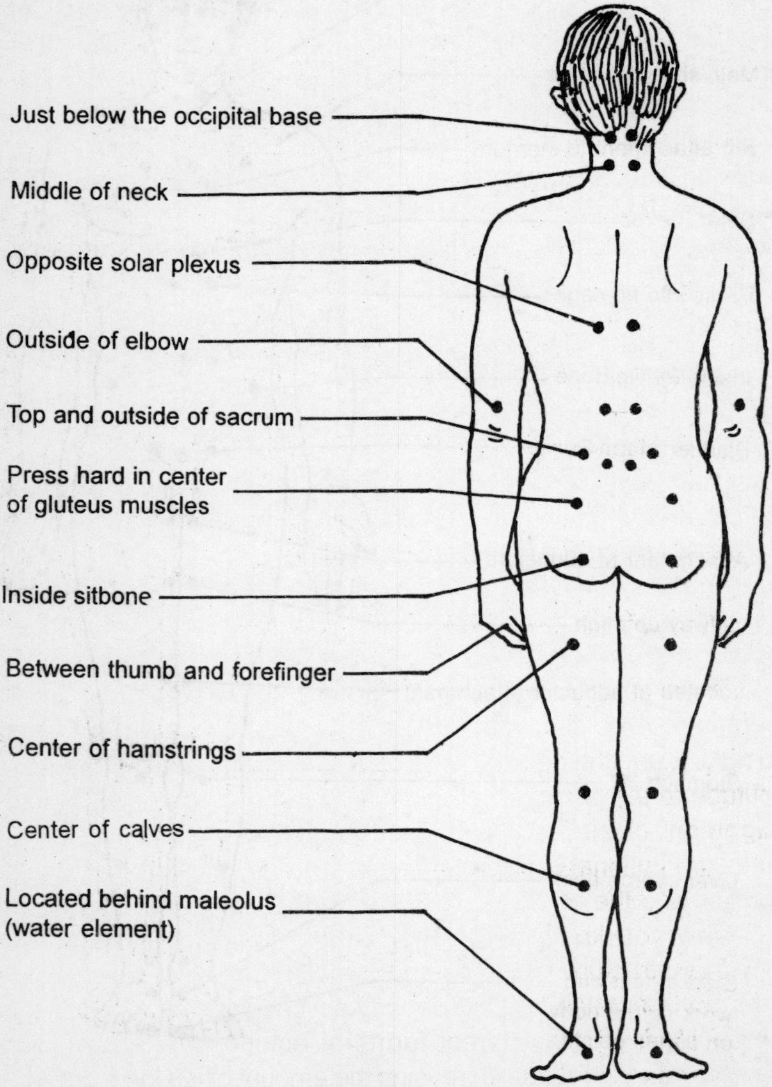

Every part of the body expresses something, according to its special body mind function. The given charts will tell you about the different types of emotions which are held in specific areas of the body. Note that there is also a definite connection between the chakras or seven main energy centers, and the types of emotions that are stored in the corresponding areas of the body. Just as the endocrine system corresponds directly to the chakras, or energy centers, the Mental and Emotional Bodies are also closely linked similarly.

Our body is a true expression of the mind and emotions. In addition to factors such as heredity, environment, nutritions, and daily physical activity, the powerful emotions and thought forms which move through the body help to mould its posture and structure.

What kind of physical structure can be called ideal?

A person with a healthy body/mind structure, when standing upright will show upon examination that his or her ears are directly above the shoulders, the shoulders are centered over the hips, the hips are directly over the knees and the knees over the ankles. If any of these areas are out of alignment, we can readily begin to note certain inferences about the person's character type or personality.

The emotional as well as physical traumas cause tightening and rigidification of the muscular and myofacial tissues of the body. Fear, grief and anger, as they pass through the body, would cause the muscles to flex in certain "protective" postures. If the person repeats these postures several times, they would begin to rigidify, and the person would then start to assume the physical attitude to the particular emotion. When they occur, the natural alignment of the body is disrupted, and an overall inflexibility and, gravitational imbalance sets in. This way, a habit pattern is formed and the physical problems appear.

Now you know about the certain common divisions in physical structure which seem to occur often, and which help simplify the understanding of body psychology.

In most of the different forms of emotional release work healers concentrate on increasing the amount of life force energy in order to push up against any blocked channels in the subtle bodies. As the life force energy comes up against a block, the resistance which occurs sets off a high pitched vibratory state in the body. All the bodily systems are in turn affected, this helps to stimulate and recreate the original trauma which created the blockage. The person then re-experiences the feelings associated with that event in the form of verbal discharge and possibly even an orgastic response. Rebirthing also employs an increase in vital energy through the vehicle of conscious breathing, in order to create the vibratory pressure needed to break through blocks for normal flow of emotions.

The different methods of emotional release work all share a common goal, which is to initiate a cathartic release of emotional energy at a level beyond the functioning of the intellectual and rational faculties. Such a release helps to purge long accumulated trauma. Technique is not necessarily an essential factor in reaching this goal, as the result is more often due to the readiness of the recipient's psyche to release such energy. A less than cathartic release where the person is still in conscious control yet is verbalizing emotion, perhaps experiencing body twitching or involuntary movements, is also helpful, as this may be the extent to which a person is prepared to release.

## FACTORS WHICH PROMOTE A SUCCESSFUL EMOTIONAL RELEASE

The healer should have a solid background in his or her technique, along with a deep understanding of the essentials of body psychology. Ideally the practitioner should acquire plenty of experience in not only helping others through release work, but also in completing a significant number of emotional clearings on oneself. In other words, in order to relate properly and create the feeling of a safe environment for cathartic release, there needs to be an empathetic sense of trust and security between both the healer and healee.

There are various techniques which help to promote a pressurized, high vibratory rate for intense emotional release. Such tools as conscious breathing, pressure points on certain parts of the body, visualization, and exercises such as those in Bioenergetics all help to move energy.

Reiki is often used in conjunction with Rebirthing. Another powerful tool to add to these two are pressure points on the body.

Some Reiki Masters utilize conscious breathing as the main tool for regression, they generally give a brief overview of body psychology and encourage the participants to evaluate each other. Bodies are examined to determine where each individual is holding the most energy and just what pressure point might help to release the blockage. If you wish to do the same. Take the time to evaluate your body with the help of somebody. Try to examine which areas have the most blockage and determine which emotional release points would have the greatest effect on your particular body type. You may refer to diagrams as guide to acquire the help of a professional rebirther/body worker and discuss your particular holding areas, and the present issue you would like to examine which is most affecting your life. With the use of conscious breathing you can then help guide your rebirther into specific pressure points in your body. After you have become familiar with the rebirthing process, you can begin to rebirth yourself. You can utilize the following technique on yourself as stated by giving instructions to an assistant.

It would be better to use most of the pressure point shown in the diagrams by starting at the feet and moving slowly up the body. Always exert pressure gently as the healee inhales, and maintain pressure or loosen if necessary on the exhale. As you come to important blockage point, you might try to exert a bit more pressure, yet at the same time, be sure that pressure does not build up to the point that it cannot get through the narrowed channel. Keep the energy flowing around the block and move back and forth on the body as necessary. Allow the energy to move, do not force it. When certain areas are not flowing, focus on the main pressure points in that area, such as the pelvis and thigh for the leg, or the shoulder for the arm.

Do not talk too much unless appropriate. Engaging the intellect tends to detract from the process. Wait until the emotions have been released before asking too many questions. As the energy moves through the body you may note certain symptoms such as twitching, spasms, etc. The healee may even cry when energy is released in the throat chakra. Allow the energy to take it's natural course. If an intense cathartic reaction occurs and you are acting as the guide, be sure to stay very grounded and focus on protecting the person from bodily harm or prolonged withholding of the breath. There is little or no facilitating needed at this point. Your intuition will tell you when the process has ended, or the healee will begin to engage in conscious interaction. After the emotional release is complete, you may want to share your experience with your rebirther, or if you are acting as the facilitator, you should allow your client to talk about his or her experience.

The emotional release work is a powerful tool for cleansing the energy body, however it does not help to reprogram ingrained habits which are associated with the release. To re-educate old subconscious patterns, try a 40-day programme of affirmations which deal directly with the issue or issues which have been released. It takes at least 40 days to reprogramme the subconscious, thus a 15-minute per day meditation utilizing appropriate affirmations is recommended for your client.

# WHEN REIKI SEEMS INEFFECTIVE

People working as Reiki healers sometimes notice that the results they expect, do not always occur. Why?

One of the reason behind it may well be something which is not immediately apparent. Every client does not like to talk about his inner life and important changes often start to take place on this level. Frequently, the patient himself has no clear idea of what has been going on within him, and it may take weeks or even months before the effects of such a treatment can be noticed.

Do not get disheartened if your expectations are not fulfilled immediately. With Reiki, nothing is to be achieved by pure willpower. Healer's egos have to take second place instead, which is not bad for his development. As Reiki channel, healer does not do the healing himself but is simply a neutral observer and witness of events. For this reason, the healer should never disapprove of a patient's symptoms. It is not his task to fight against an illness but to pass on Reiki energy and await the results, which will always be satisfactory.

There are some interesting reasons why Reiki sometimes fails to work. For example, healer would have experienced again and again that, although patients come for treatment, the willingness to be healed is simply an alibi. In their innermost beings such patients, consciously or unconsciously, do not want to be made healthy again. On the contrary, they cling to their illnesses, which are obviously advantageous to them in some way. There was once a retired person, for example, who only got the support and affection of his family when he was ill. This was probably the only way he had. When this kind of experience is deeply rooted, the patient will probably have an inner resistance to any kind of treatment that could help him. Of course, on the outside it will look as if he has done everything he could to become healthy again; no stone has been left unturned, and even a new and popular method has been tried.

A similar phenomenon can be discovered in the case of some neglected children, but not generally to such a marked degree. When a child is ill, he or she is given extra attention and generally shown a lot of love and sympathy. He or she will not have to go to school, and everyone will be generally nice to him or her. When such a child has balanced out what it had been previously lacking, it will then, but only then, find it easy to become healthy again. This mechanism is generally an unconscious one, and we should not feel bad when a child seems to be taking advantage of the situation.

Sometimes we also act in this manner. For weeks or months we overdo things, and then, when we can no longer go on, we become ill, gaining the peace and quiet we had not been granting ourselves as well as the care and attention of our loved ones, which we had not been getting, in a way which is generally accepted. After all, a sick person is sympathized with, for it is not his fault for getting ill at exactly that moment in time. And once he gets better, everything will seem to be in order once again.

Besides that there are other reasons for Reiki apparently failing to have the desired effect. It once happened that a man did not return after he had been treated for the first time, which puzzled the healer very much. He then found out from his sister that he had experienced Reiki as being something strange and dubious, nobody knows why he reacted in that way, but there are people who have never encountered spiritual things before and who prefer something more sound than Reiki.

Hence, never persuade someone to let himself be treated with Reiki. Instead, simply tell him what Reiki is and how it works and leave the decision up to him. This will generally lead to satisfactory treatment. Another reason for Reiki apparently failing to work might be that the person involved has not yet learned the lesson taught by the illness and that he therefore has to go on being ill for a little while. On the other hand, illness may prevent a person from repeatedly breaking laws of nature and doing damage to himself, in which case Reiki treatment could well open up such a patient's eyes to the inner causes of his condition. In this case, the patient suddenly becomes aware of why he or she is ill and starts to change things on an inner and outer level.

There is also the kind of patient who finds Reiki too simple. Such patients are afraid that people will think they had not really been ill if they could be cured so easily. They prefer hospitals, expensive nursing homes, etc.

Then there are those who come for treatment in order to prove to you and themselves that a method like Reiki cannot possibly have any effect whatsoever. They lie on the treatment table full of tension and scepticism, resisting every flow of energy and every kind of pleasant feeling and fighting the possibility of inner change occurring and harmony setting in. Some of them will manage to remain as they were before treatment.

Hence, when someone comes to you for treatment, provide him with information and offer him the possibility of treatment but do not press it on him. Each person has his own free will, and a wise healer should respect this.

These kind of things do not occur very often and their existence should not prevent healer from approaching each new case in an unbiased way.

You will definitely experience very wonderful cures with Reiki, although the way they come about will sometimes surprise you. Simply remain open for Life Force Energy.

# REIKI IN THE EVOLUTION OF CONSCIOUSNESS

Many circumstances are providing people with an opportunity to wake up to become more consciously aware, and to begin to break out of the mould of race mind consciousness. The old denial patterns and fears, which have been passed down for centuries from generation to generation, are slowly disappearing as we begin to sense the new vibratory frequency of love in our world and adjust ourselves accordingly to it. We can no longer separate ourselves from each other and survive. We have created a situation where we must choose to cooperate or die. The old unconscious pattern of separation is fading away as we move towards a new collective consciousness of peace and harmony for the mankind.

All discomfort is caused by negative emotions, due to a basic guilt of separation from God by a false ego, unhappy feelings of frustration. If one can for a moment escape the self-centered ego which always makes people restless, one may become aware that we are not separated from God (our true-self and the true-selves of others); that indeed we truly are at one with the Universe (not separate). Through such a recognition, all blessings are bestowed. Healing occurs through remembrance. Indeed, remembering who we truly are is the key to self-healing. Remembering where our emotions first got out of hand and react on the physical body is another important clue to discovering our specific misunderstandings which also relate back to the initial feeling of separateness. A quantum leap in the consciousness of mankind is now needed to defeat this old feeling of separation and neglect.

Reiki is a powerful medium which can help the individual release this sense of separation. As the 21-day cleanse process commences after the First Degree Class, many old emotional blocks begin to be released. Intuition also becomes heightened, helping the individual to become more finely tuned to the higher self and attain enlightenment.

By amplifying the vibratory rate of the body, Reiki enables each person to channel larger amounts of energy, and also raises the vibratory level of the planet as a whole.

Reiki is also a tool of empowerment, it provides each individual with an opportunity to strip away the veils over consciousness which tend to hinder a clear perception of truth. As we seek through inner work to develop greater conscious awareness, and a deeper level of communication with the Higher Self, we will see the resulting effect of these veils being lifted.

# ETHICS OF PROFESSION

* Dr. Usui said that never give away the Reiki, it makes beggars of the people you give it to. Remember, though, that the exchange can take many forms.

* One should never diagnose or prescribe unless he is licensed to do so (i.e.., an M.D., Chiropractor, Acupuncturist, D.O., etc.).

* Never try to go beyond the limits of what you are trained to do (i.e., only do massage if you are trained in massage, and never do counselling unless you are trained in that).

* The information given to you by your Reiki clients should remain confidential.

* Never touch anybody inappropriately.

* One should never take advantage of the bond that develops between him and the client whom he is treating. If you are treating someone in a therapeutic setting, it is inappropriate to date or have sexual relations with him or her.

* You are not supposed to heal the whole world. You do not have to treat everyone. If it doesn't feel right to treat someone, don't treat.

* Be accurate and honest, accurate in the way you present yourself to the public regarding your level of Reiki training.

* One should always use common sense when doing Reiki.

* One should be fully dressed and the clothing should be appropriate when doing a treatment. Many Reiki people prefer all-natural fibres because they tend to absorb any perspiration created. Reiki is accepted or rejected at the soul level of the receiver. Your job is to be there; the rest is up to them. This holds true for whatever level of Reiki you are working with.

* Undressing is not necessary for a Reiki treatment. Do not have your client disrobe unless you are doing something in addition to Reiki, such as massage (and if you have a licence for that).

* Never think that you have magical powers or you are doing the healing. Reiki does the healing, you are only a link.

# TEMPTATIONS

You will be tempted at every step of your life. Temptation is also a part of spiritual growth. The temptations are there for you to overcome and grow by, not to be hung up in and wallow in. You will also be tempted by what you are most temptable with: if ice-cream is your weakness, you won't be tempted with vegetable soup. Whatever temptations you have already worked through will not need to come up for you again in this lifetime, unless of course there are other and probably deeper levels yet to be conquered. Reiki often helps speed up this process.

It is wise to have a few friends you can count on who are willing to be totally, honest. When you are being challenged by one of the temptations you will almost assuredly not be able to see it for yourself. This is when you will need your friends, willing and able to confront you on what they see. Confront is what they will probably have to do, because what you are into will seem absolutely right to you. But your honest friends can tell you exactly what they feel about following :

**GREED**
**EGO**
**PRIDE**
**HUNGER FOR POWER**

The awareness of temptations, be it now or later, makes it easier on a daily basis to really look at what is going on in your life. Newcomers usually ask what the specific temptations will be once they start on a Reiki path. The temptations will show up in all areas of your life; with respect to Reiki, usually they will have something to do with wanting to be a Reiki Master, or with thinking you are doing the healing rather than the Reiki energy doing the healing, hence, that makes you superior than the patient.

**Greed:** might lead you to believe you can be a Reiki Master without paying $10,000 Dr. Hayashi set as its value.

**Ego:** might make you feel that you, not Reiki, is doing the healing.

**Pride:** might force you to think that you deserve the title of Reiki Master and that you, not your Master, are the one to decide this.

**Hunger for Power:** might make you think you should be superior than other humans, and be stronger in your Reiki than they are.

Remember that the higher you go on a spiritual path the harder the lessons get. Some think the lessons should get easier, but they do not, that is how we grow. Remember that we all have free will and are never forced into any growth we do not want. Avoid temptation to achieve better results.

# LEGAL ASPECTS

What one needs to do to a Reiki practice? It depends on the legal requirements of the place you want to practice. When you finish a Reiki class you get a certificate. That is totally different from getting a license to charge money for treatment. Licenses are given primarily by government bodies of towns or cities. In some states licence is not required. But you must confirm it before starting Reiki practice.

You must be legal if you are going to charge money from the client. If you are giving treatments to your family and friends the legal requirements are looser, besides, of course, general decency and the patient's consent. If, however, you wish to work on the public, make sure you abide by whatever laws are in force in the area in which you wish to practice.

In Eastern countries where Reiki originated, the laws regarding where you can place your hands on another person are quite different from the laws in the Western countries. One should try to keep the Reiki technique pure, however it is extremely important that when doing Reiki you are ethical in all that you do at all times. This is far more important than abiding by the hand positions which were taught previously.

# PRINCIPLES OF GENERAL TREATMENT

**Law of Opposites** is commonly used in acupuncture. These principles may be used alone or in conjunction with local treatment.

1. Treat the opposite limb contralaterally, left arm to right leg.
2. For that which is above, treat that which is below. For instance, treat the abdomen in cases of headaches.
3. Treat the opposite limb, leg to leg or arm to arm.
4. Treat same side arm and leg.

Law of opposites also applies to the front and back of the torso. For example, In a backache, by treating the corresponding area on the front you may achieve better results.

**Organ Clock** of the Chinese gives you ideas as to where to concentrate for treatment, based on the time of day.

| | |
|---|---|
| 11 am to 1 pm is Heart | 11 pm to 1 am is Gall bladder |
| 11 pm to 3 pm is Small Intestine | 1 am to 3 am is Liver |
| 3 pm to 5 pm is Urinary Bladder | 3 am to 5 am is Lung |
| 5 pm to7 pm is Kidney | 5 am to 7 am is Large Intestine |
| 7 pm to 9 pm is Pericardium | 7 am to 9 am is Stomach |
| 9 pm to 11 pm is Triple Warmer | 9 am to 11 am is Spleen/ Pancreas |

The Triple Warmer is sometimes thought of as the connective tissue surrounding the abdominal cavity.

Though, according to some healers some of these times are not convenient. Through the law of opposites, they treat an organ energy which is active from 3 am to 5 am during the afternoon between 3 pm and 5 pm. In other words, they treat for the lung during the bladder time.

# POSITIONS OF HANDS

The hand positions given in this chapter are changed slightly, because the laws in the Orient tend to be very different from Western laws regarding such issues as touching another individual. Many of the original hand positions taught for treating another person with Reiki are illegal in many countries. Using the new hand positions shown in this manual will give you the same results as the classical positions, while remaining legally and ethically appropriate.

This comprehensive manual is a result of the vast new levels of knowledge the Reiki teachers have gained over the last 15 years regarding how Reiki works. This manual is for the layman as well as both beginning and advanced Reiki practitioners.

For each of the hand positions of a classical treatment as much information is covered as possible regarding the way Reiki works to enhance physical, mental, emotional and spiritual balancing, as well as its effect on the Chakras.

To start the ideal classical treatment you should start with **Head Position 1** and go straight through to **Back Position 6,** spending about 3 minutes in each position. In all hand positions, the fingers are kept gently together, and, whenever possible, touching at the midline of the body.

Ideal classical treatment takes about 60 to 90 minutes. Realistically, many treatments are done on the run with far less time than this to complete them, so there are various ways to do Reiki treatment. You can do a full treatment, or a short treatment, or treat where it pains or put your hands on the client.

## HEAD * * * * * * * * * * * * *POSITIONS-1

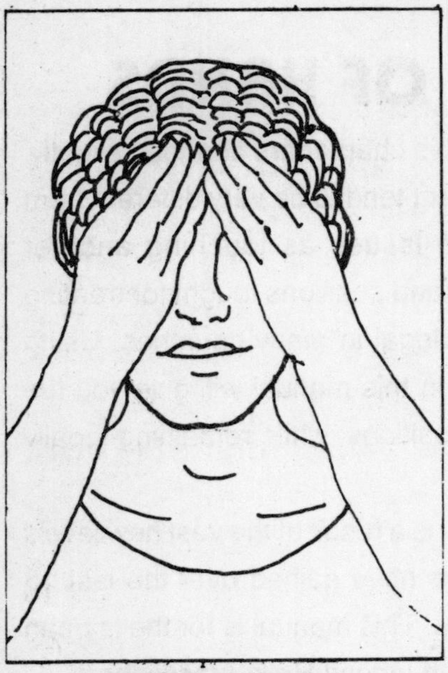

Self-Treatment

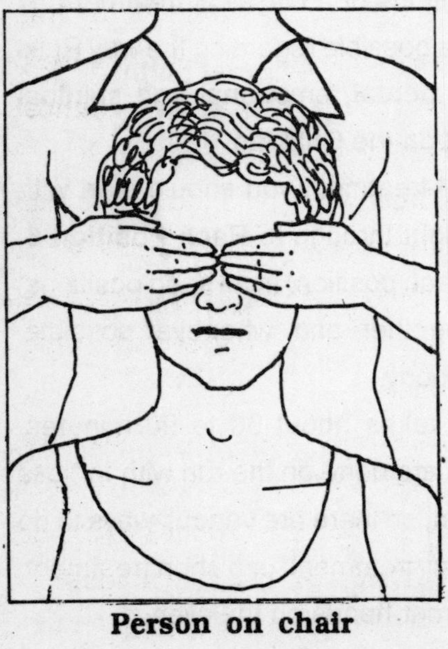

Person on chair

**The Chakra**

Third Eye

**Oriental Faith**

The third eye is the center of such forms of extra-sensory perception like clairvoyance and telepathy. It is here where we visualize things, because it is the seat of will, spirit and the intellect. Treatment of this area enhances clairvoyance which is clear seeing. Sinus cavity congestion can block the senses like sight, taste and scent, etc. which are associated with this position.

**Physical Features**

Eyes and any condition relating to eyes—nearsightedness, far sightedness, glaucoma, detached retina, cataract, etc.

- Headaches, colds & flu, sinuses,
- Pineal and pituitary glands,
- Teeth,
- Jaws-TMJ (temporo mandibular joint dysfunctions)

**Mental & Emotional Features**

- Relaxation and stress reduction,

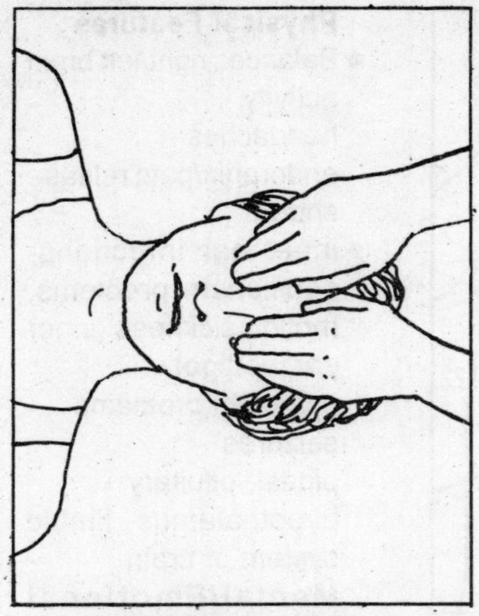

**Person on table**

clarity in one's life,

- Vision or ability to see what is needed-relationships, changes, career, etc.

**Spiritual Features**

- Meditation,
- Help to get centered-explore oneself,
- Activation of internal light i.e., flashes of light, pictures of past lives or current events, kaleidoscopes of colours, etc.

## Positions of Hands

In this, both hands should be placed gently over the eyes.

## HEAD * * * * * * * * * * * *POSITIONS-2

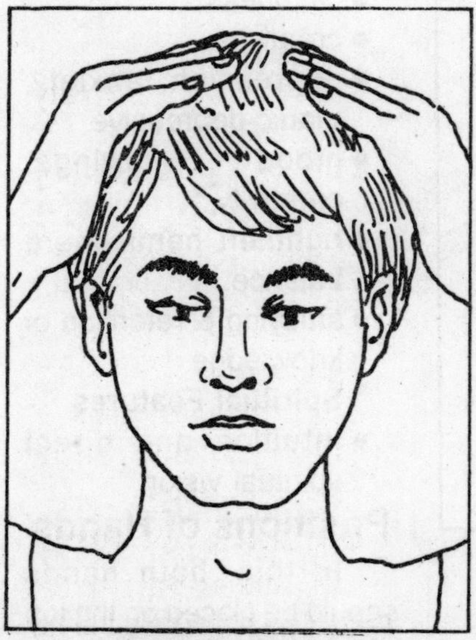

**Self-Treatment**

**The Chakra**

Crown Chakra or Lotus Chakra

**Oriental Faith**

This crown center represents the highest level of consciousness that mankind can attain. The balancing of the right and left brain takes place here. A place of divine inspiration. The universal healing power of Reiki transmits to the whole organism through the vascular, neurological and energetic conduits finding their meeting place here.

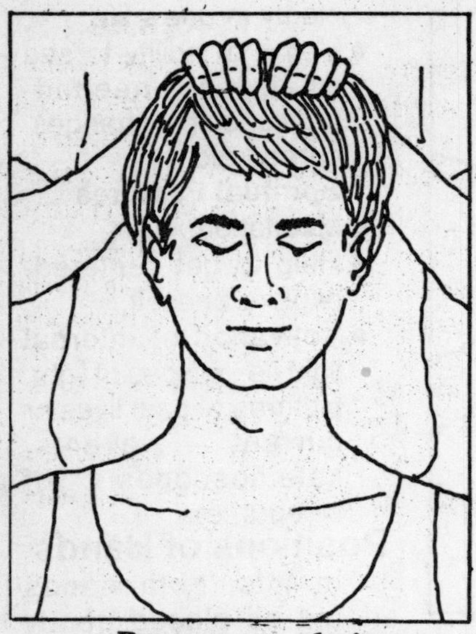

Person on chair

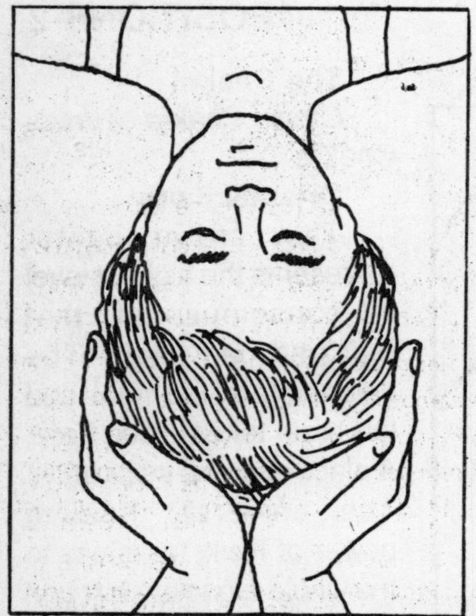

Person on table

**Physical Features**

- Balances right/left brain activity, headaches endorphin/pain release shock
- inner ear infections-equilibrium problems, motion sickness (inner ear, vertigo), eye stem problems seizures pineal, pituitary hypothalamus, limbic system of brain

**Mental/Emotional Features**

- Balancing mental/emotional problems
- memory
- calmness
- creativity
- depression, anxiety, manic-depressive,
- mood swings, creativity,
- right/left hemisphere balance,
- studying & retention of knowledge

**Spiritual Features**

- Intuition and direct spiritual vision.

## Positions of Hands

In this, both hands should be placed on the top of head with fingers or side of hands touching

## HEAD * * * * * * * * * * * * * * *POSITIONS-3

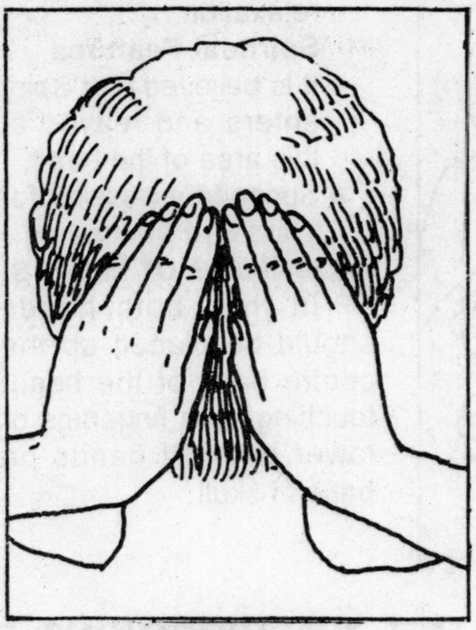

**Self-Treatment**

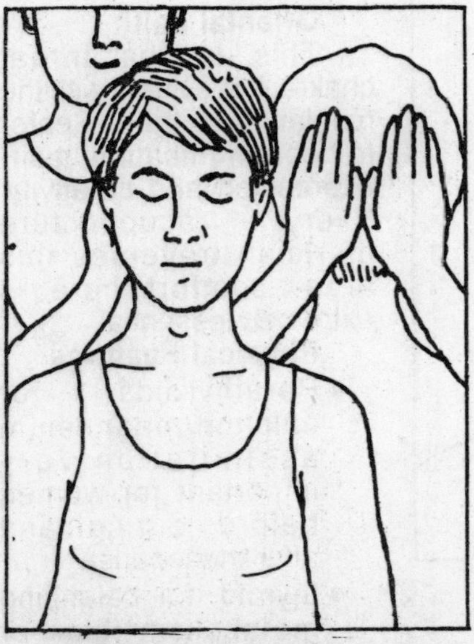

**Person on chair**

**Oriental Faith**

Situated in the lower brain stem, this area addresses unconscious urges and patterns. Use this area to treat addictive behavioural patterns. This area is stimulated by the Rosicrucians to generate a state of wakefulness and mindfulness. The lower brain stem is also considered as an essential link to the greater beingness.

**Physical Features**

- Treats old brain/ reptilian brain,
- treats back of eye stem,
- more left/right hemisphere balancing,
- more inner ear,
- governs basic bodily functions, commands heart to beat, lungs to breathe, food to digest, etc.
- asthma, pneumonia, various heart/ circulatory problems, sleep disorders.

**Mental/Emotional Features**

- pituitary and pineal (balancing of the glands),
- past life and past dream recall,

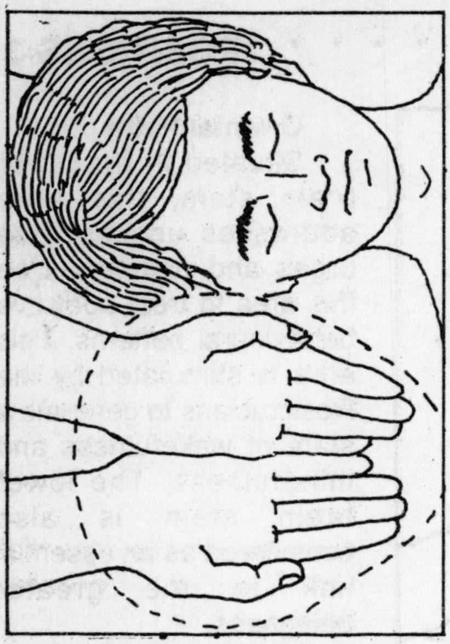

Person on table

- very nurturing position for self/others relaxation.

**Spiritual Features**

- It is believed that Spirit enters and leaves at this area of the head,
- Secondary position for Third Eye treatment,

## Positions of Hands

In this, both hands should be placed up the centre back of the head, touching, with fingertips or lower palm of hands on base of skull

## HEAD * * * * * * * * * * * *POSITIONS-4

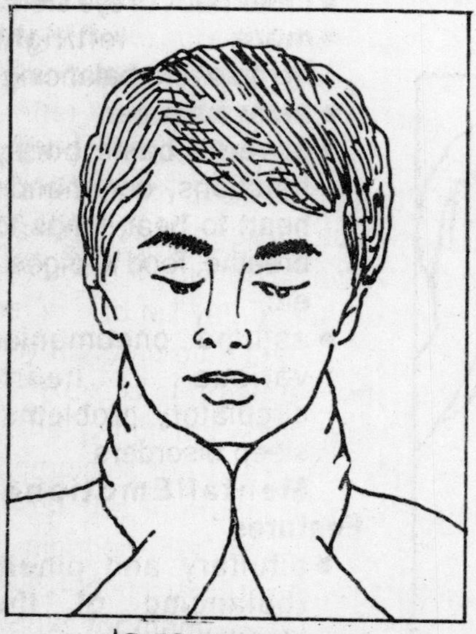

Self-Treatment

**The Chakra**

Throat

**Oriental Faith**

This is the throat chakra. It is evident with the revelation of truth. Center for communication, self-expression and creativity. Every acupuncture meridian traverses this area; comfort here is extremely essential.

**Physical Features**

- Parathyroids for calcium/magnesium assimilation-very important for women before, during, and after menopause,
- thyroid, for balancing metabolism (high or low),

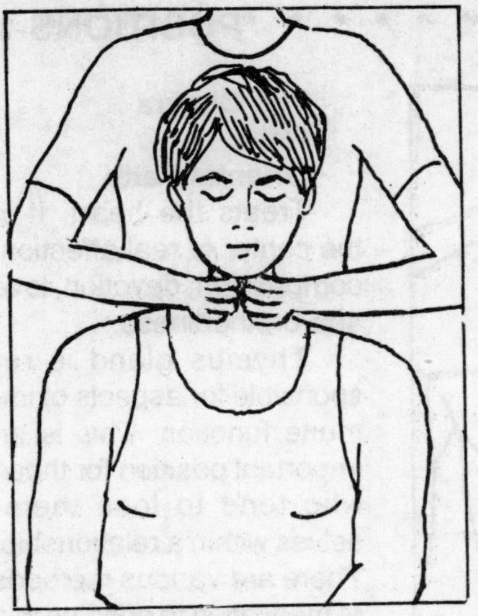

**Person on chair**

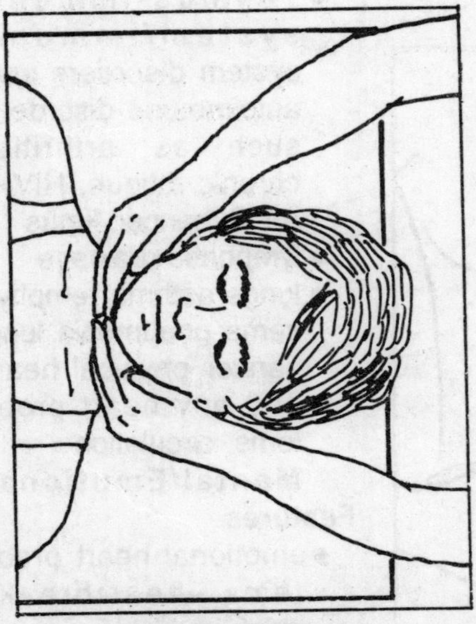

**Person on table**

- lymphatic drainage,
- osteoporosis,
- carotid artery for treating blood, especially blood entering brain,
- balances high or low blood pressure,
- haemoglobin/hematocrit,
- circulation
- strokes
- believed to be effective in assisting medications which cross blood/brain barrier
- might affect balancing medications,
- tonsillitis, sore throat, larynx,

**Mental/Emotional Features**

- major power center for the body; control by tone of voice and spoken words, codependency recovery because of power/control issues,
- especially important for anger and rage,
- self-confidence, anxiety, stage fright-particularly pertinent for performers, self-confidence
- communication
- stabilizing

## Positions of Hands

In this, both hands should be placed gently on the throat with fingertips, or base of palms touching over the thyroid.

## FRONT * * * * * * * * * * * * * POSITIONS-1

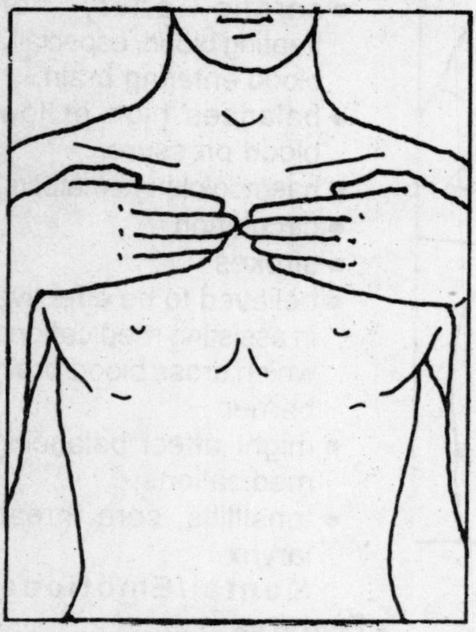

Self-Treatment

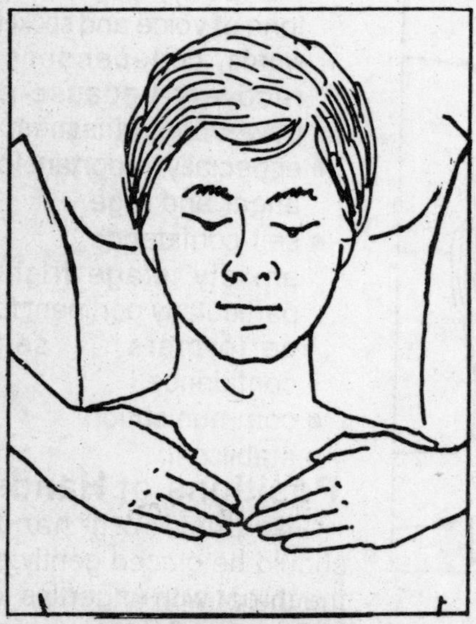

Person on chair

**The Chakra**

Heart

**Oriental Faith**

Treats the heart. It is the center of real affection, compassion, devotion, love and brotherliness.

Thymus gland is responsible for aspects of immune function. This is an important position for those who tend to lose themselves within a relationship. There are various methods of meditation to open up this Chakra.

**Physical Features**

- Thymus-immune system/immune system disorders and autoimmune disorders such as arthritis, chronic fatigue, HIV+, AIDS, cancer, lupus
- lymphatic drainage
- lungs asthma, emphysema, pneumonia, lung cancer physical heart and any heart problems, circulation

**Mental/Emotional Features**

- emotional heart problems—heartbreak, grief, joy.
- going within
- comforting

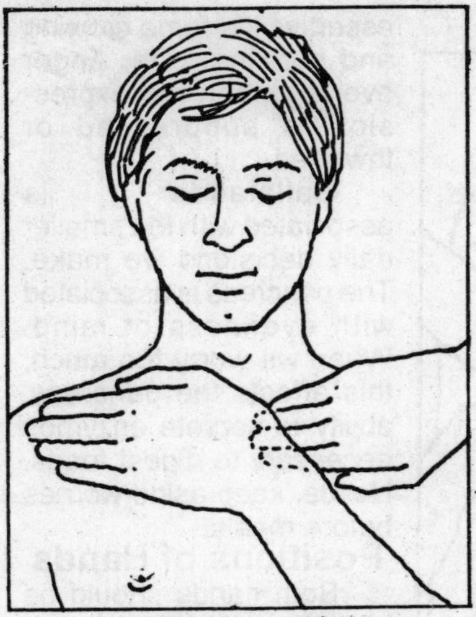

**Person on table**

- balancing any strong feelings
- entering, returning to self

**Spiritual Features**

- believed to be the location that the spirit leaves the body at the moment of death.
- unconditional love
- compassion
- devotion

## Positions of Hands

In this, both hands are placed on the upper chest over the thymus with the fingers touching

## FRONT * * * * * * * * * * * POSITIONS-2&3

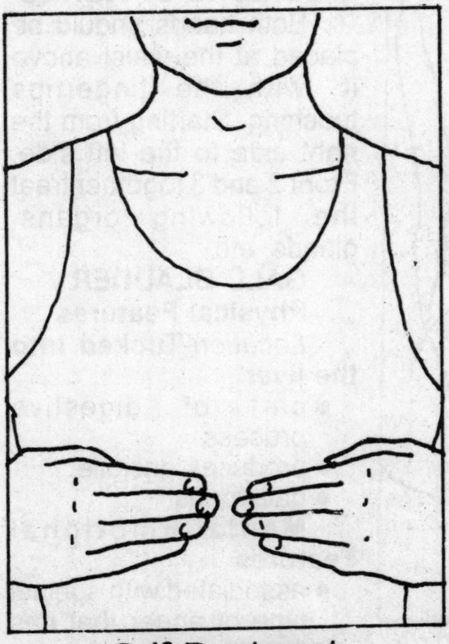

**Self-Treatment**

**The Chakra**

Spleen

**Oriental Faith**

Treats the solar plexus. The place where physical energy is distributed. Organs situated here are the liver, spleen, gallbladder and pancreas.

Spleen is a large lymph node which filters blood and lymph. This position is one of the most important for daily physical well-being, including the diaphragm, many important organs are situated here.

The emotion associated with the liver and gallbladder is anger. When naturally expressed, it is an

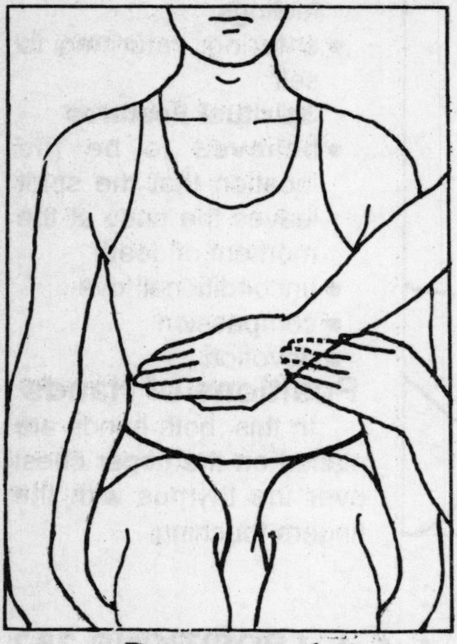
Person on chair

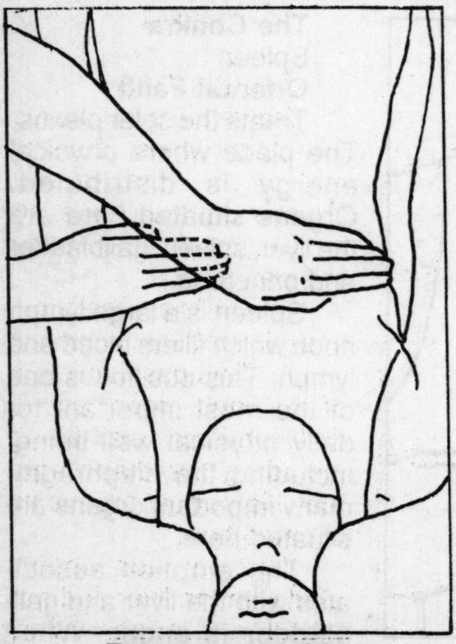
Person on table

assertive life force growing and bursting forth. Anger evolves when the expression is suppressed or thwarted.

Gallbladder is associated with the smaller daily decisions we make. The pancreas is associated with evenness of mind. When we worry too much, this affects the pancreas' ability to secrete enzymes necessary to digest foods. Hence, keep aside worries before meals.

## Positions of Hands

Both hands should be placed under the chest, over the rib cage with fingertips touching at the base of the chestbone

## Positions of Hands

Both hands should be placed at the waist above it, with the fingertips touching. Starting from the right side to the left side, Front 2 and 3 together treat the following organs, glands, etc.

**GALL BLADDER**

**Physical Features**

*Location*-**Tucked into the liver**

- part of digestive process
- produces gall/bile
- gallstones

**Mental/Emotional Features**

- associated with special type of anger that has bitterness to it
- decision-making organ

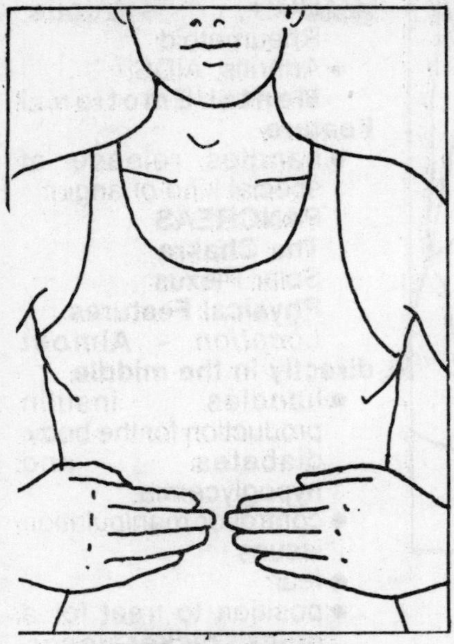

**Self-Treatment**

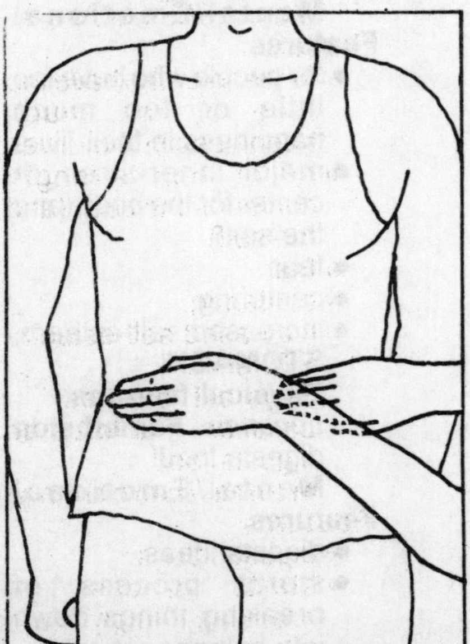

**Person on chair**

**LIVER**

**Physical Features**

*Location* - **Far right side**

- primary organ for detox-not just alcohol, which is processed in the liver, but any other toxin as well, such as, the pesticides/ insecticides that our food has been treated with, the chemicals present in the air we breathe and the water we drink.
- headaches,
- hormonal imbalances such as PMS in women & midlife crisis in men,
- estrogen metabolized in liver,
- processes medications
- metabolizes lactic acid
- cholesterol
- environmental allergies
- jaundice

**Mental/Emotional Features**

- emotionally, liver is unresolved anger issues processing old issues/feelings

**SPLEEN**

**Physical Features**

*Location* - **Behind the stomach**

- blood purifier—treat here for any infections anywhere in the body,
- manufactures T-cells and is extremely important for treatment of any immune system disorders,
- also important for autoimmune disorders

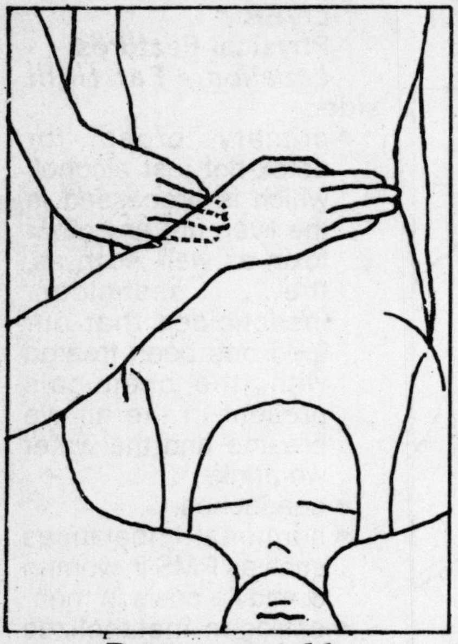

Person on table

such as: chronic fatigue,

- Epstein-Barr Virus, HIV+, Lupus, Rheumatoid
- Arthritis, AIDS

**Mental/Emotional Feature**

- handles release of special kind of anger.

**PANCREAS**

**The Chakra**

Solar Plexus

**Physical Features**

*Location* - **Almost directly in the middle**

- handles insulin production for the body, diabetes and hypoglycemia
- control or manipulation issues
- fear
- position to treat for a quick picker-upper, when energy is low

**Mental/Emotional Features**

- for people who have too little or too much happiness in their lives
- major inner-strength center for the body (and the self)
- fear
- centering
- increased self-esteem

**STOMACH**

**Physical features**

*Location* - **Far left side**

digests food

**Mental/Emotional Features**

- digests ideas,
- starts process of breaking things down into component parts,

## FRONT * * * * * * * * * * * * POSITIONS-4&5

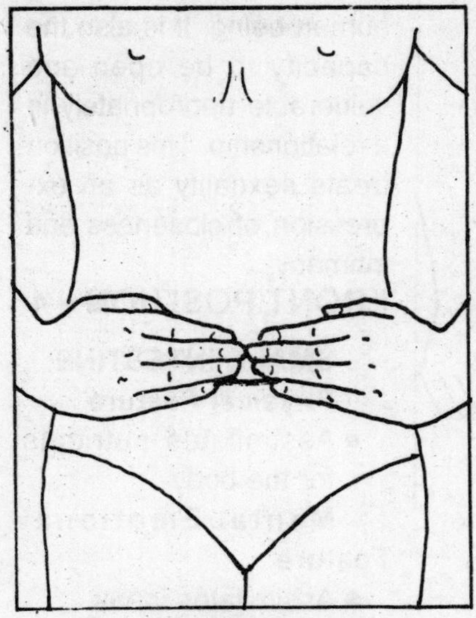

**Self-Treatment**

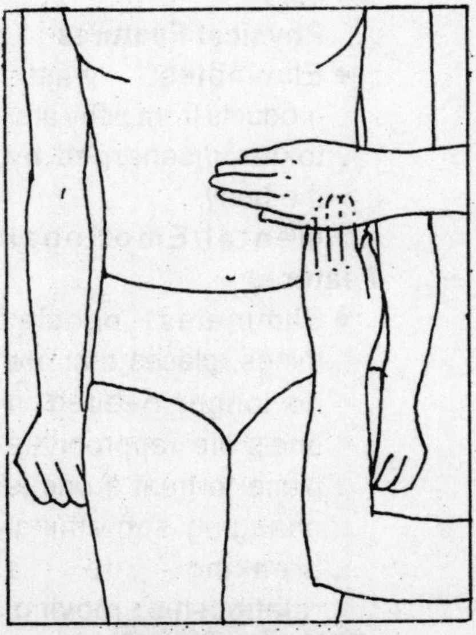

**Person on chair**

**The Chakra**

Sexual

**Oriental Faith**

This is associated with the small and large intestines. The small intestine functions to decide which nutrients we will take into our body and which ones will be left out. This also applies to other levels such as processing incoming information, experiences and emotions.

The small intestine's metaphor is sifting and processing. When there is data overload or food overload, it is easy for stagnation to take place in the small intestine.

The large intestine involves the capacity to let go of what we do not need. When free exchange of issues and things in our life is too fast, diarrhoea can result. When there is congestion in the process of letting go, constipation can be the result.

This is the second chakra, its key word is intimacy. This reflects the capacity for timely disclosure.

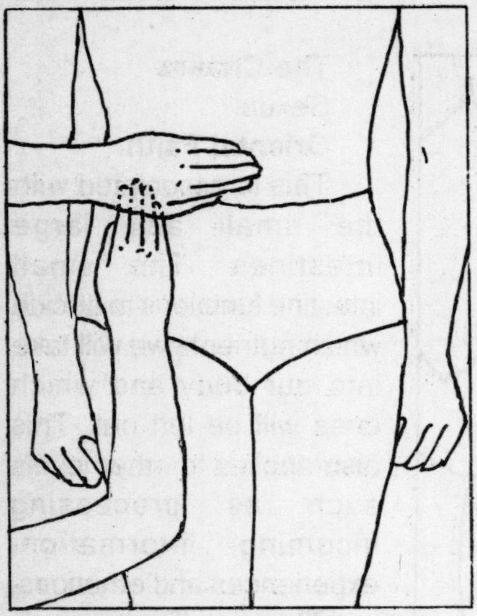

Person on table

The appropriate revelation of our story with another human being. It is also the capacity to be open and vulnerable appropriately in a relationship. This position treats sexuality as an expression of closeness and intimacy.

## FRONT POSITION—4

**SMALL INTESTINE**

**Physical Feature**

- Assimilates nutrients for the body

**Mental/Emotional Feature**

- Assimilates ideas

**LARGE INTESTINE & COLON**

**Physical Features**

- Eliminates waste products from body and toxins discharged by the body.

**Mental/Emotional Features**

- Eliminates people, things, places that are no longer needed in one's life (appropriate place to treat if one is changing something, breaking up a relationship, moving, etc.)

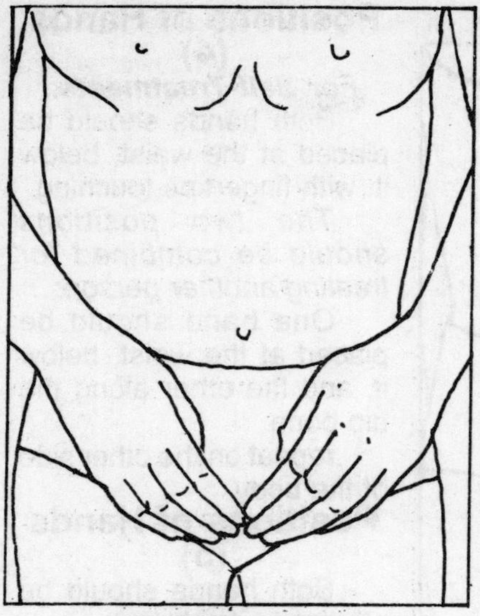

**Self-Treatment**

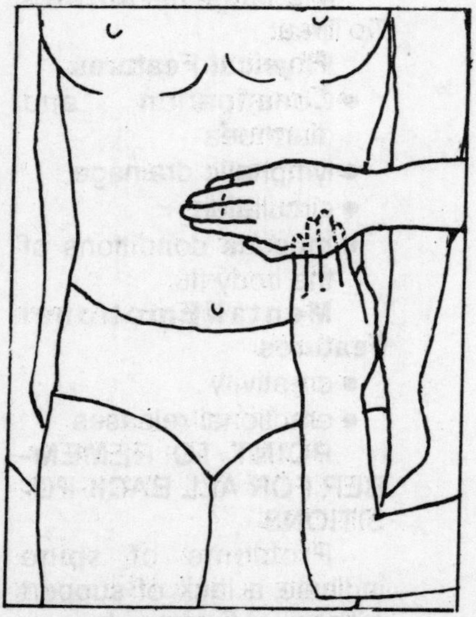

**Person on chair**

## FRONT POSITION--5

**The Chakra**

Root

**Oriental Faith**

This treats the urogenital tract and lower intestines. It is the Root Chakra. The Root Chakra is the seat of physical vitality and the fundamental urge to survive. It goes out of balance when we engage in making a living which does not match with our destiny. This Chakra revolves around the question of right livelihood.

**Physical Features**

- Female and male reproductive systems—both, and any physical or emotional problems relating to them, migraine headaches (related to sexual repression)

  bladder & its conditions

**Mental/Emotional Feature**

- Additional release (bladder)

**Spiritual Feature**

- grounding

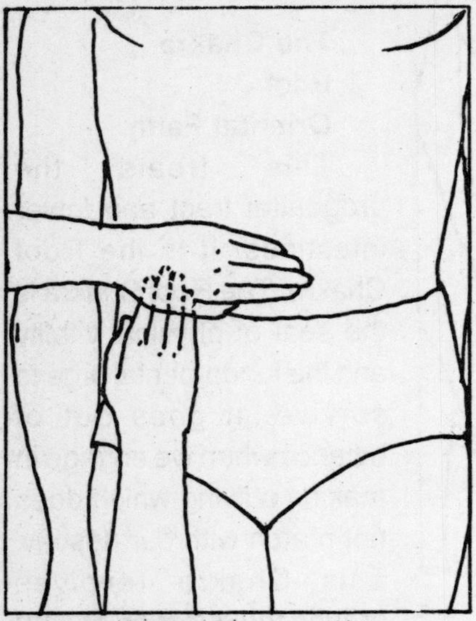

Person on table

## Positions of Hands (4)

***For Self-Treatments:***

Both hands should be placed at the waist, below it, with fingertips touching

*The two positions should be combined for treating another person:*

One hand should be placed at the waist, below it, and the other along the hip bone

repeat on the other side of the body

## Positions of Hands (5)

Both hands should be placed in such a manner that the fingertips may touch the pubic bone

4 & 5 Together Are Able To Treat:

**Physical Features**

- Constipation and diarrhoea
- lymphatic drainage
- circulation
- mucous conditions of the body flu

**Mental/Emotional Features**

- creativity
- emotional releases

**POINT TO REMEMBER FOR ALL BACK POSITIONS**

Problems of spine indicate a lack of support either financial or emotional; all back positions are quite helpful in this condition.

## BACK * * * * * * * * * * * POSITIONS-1

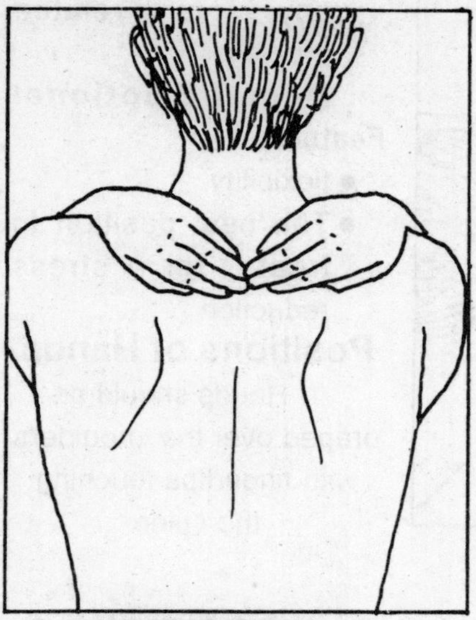

**Self–Treatment**

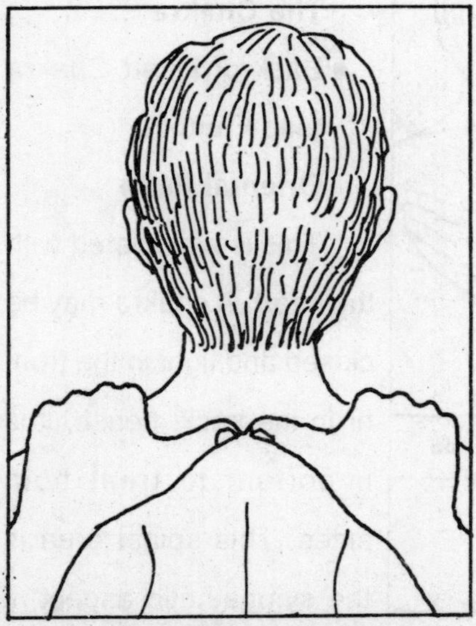

**Person on chair**

**Oriental Faith**

The Throat Chakra can be treated with this. This also stimulates and harmonizes the parasympathetic nervous system. This aspect is used for people who are nervous and tense. This position is excellent when combined with abdominal hand positions to improve digestive function through autonomic nervous system regulation. It stimulates hot bath.

**Physical Features**

- flexibility,
- starts flow of energy up/ down spine treats plexus of nerves that radiate around the heart/lung areas,
- treats spot on top of shoulders that is a major endorphin-releasing spot for the body. Endorphins are a natural morphine the body produces. Morphine kills pain, hence use this position to subdue pain

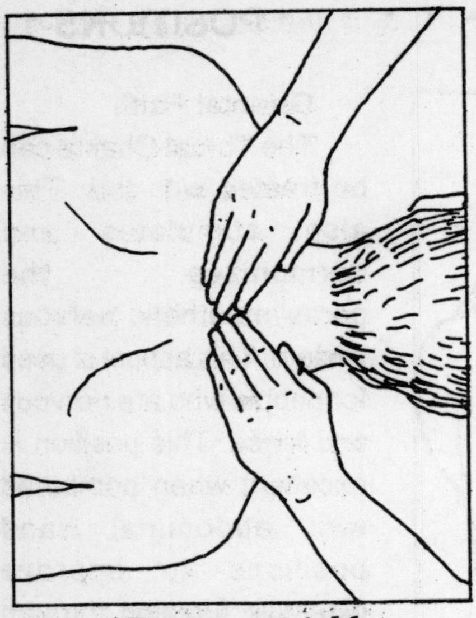

Person on table

anywhere in the body. It is also used to treat any lung-related problem

**Mental/Emotional Features**

- flexibility
- The best position to treat for stress reduction

## Positions of Hands

Hands should be draped over the shoulders with fingertips touching the spine

## BACK * * * * * * * * * * * POSITIONS-2

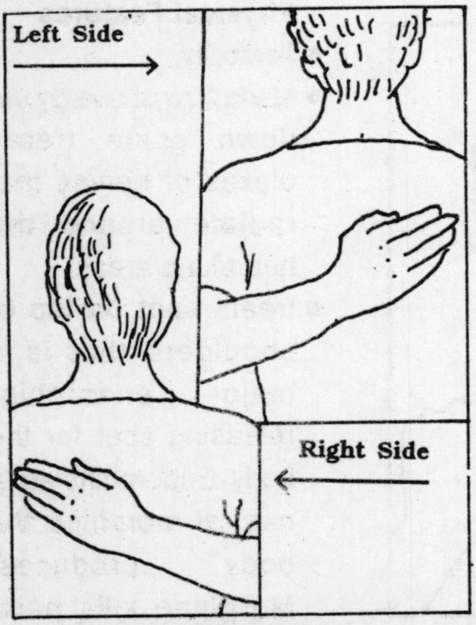


Self Treatment

**The Chakra**

- Back of Heart Chakra (see Front 1)

**Oriental Faith**

This is associated with the heart. A chakra may be closed and tight in the front or in the back, hence, it is important to treat both sides. This spinal area is the sympathetic aspect; it can be used with the rest of

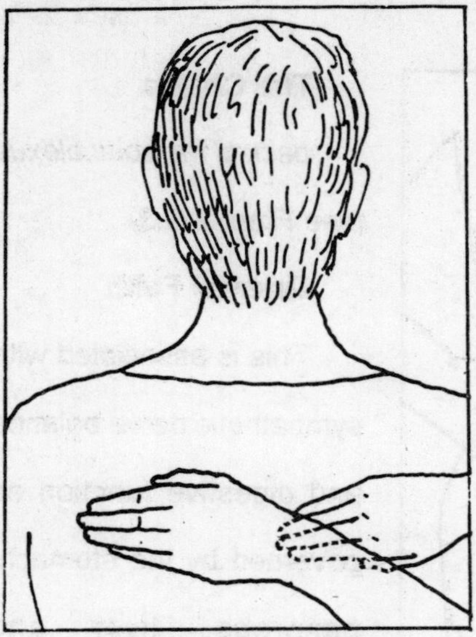

**Person on chair**

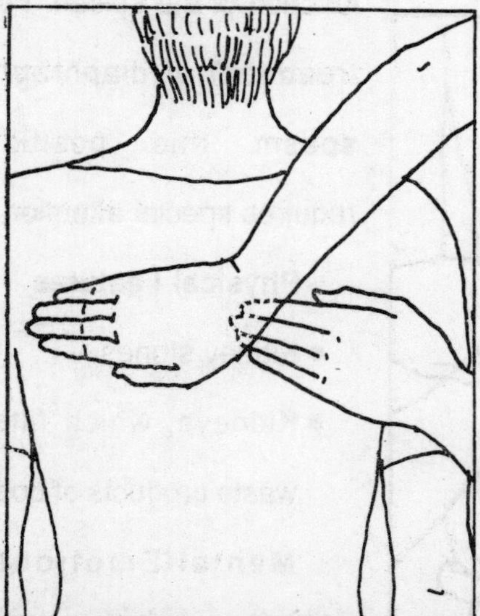

**Person on table**

the back to regulate the fight-or-flight response. This position also has acupuncture points which are used for chronic tenacious problems. This position should be used for any pattern of imbalance more than two months old.

**Physical Features**

- Back of heart, back of lungs and more of the spine

**Mental/Emotional Feature**

- Softening of rigidity as far as love is concerned

**Spiritual Feature**

- Treat here to develop the feeling of universal love

## Positions of Hands

Hands should be placed across the shoulder blades with hands touching the spine

## BACK * * * * * * * * * * POSITIONS-3

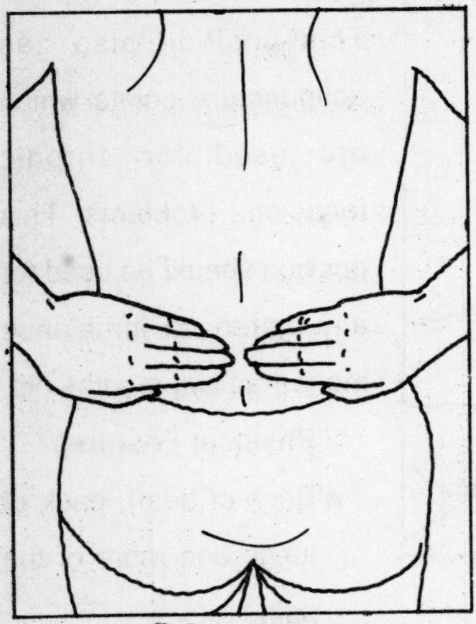

Self-Treatment

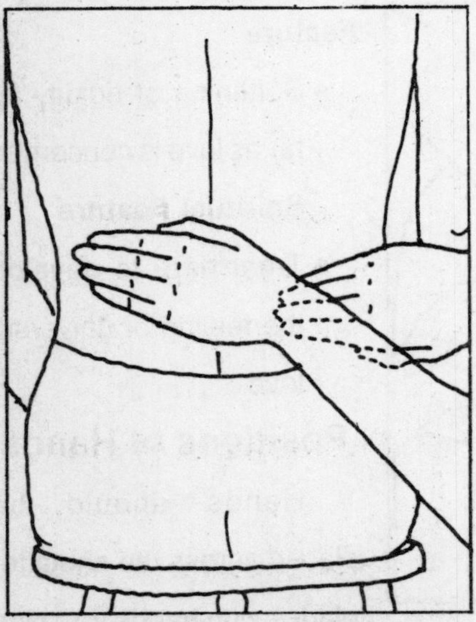

Person on chair

**The Chakra**

*back of the solar plexus*

*(see Front 2 & 3)*

**Oriental Faith**

This is associated with sympathetic nerve balance and digestive function as governed by the stomach, pancreas, liver and gallbladder. It also adjusts function of the spleen. For treatment of diaphragm spasm this position requires special attention.

**Physical Features**

- Kidney stones
- Kidneys, which filter waste products of body

**Mental/Emotional Features**

- Filter ideas and

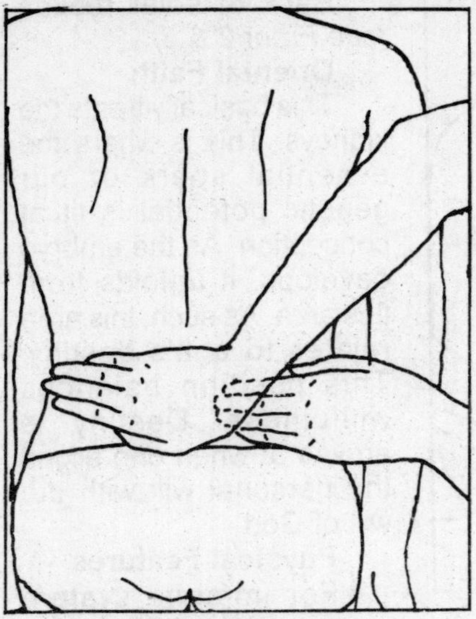

**Person on table**

concepts that are no longer useful, the kind of anger you feel when you are ditched.

## Positions of Hands

Both hands should be placed at the waist, above it, with hands touching

## BACK * * * * * * * * * * * POSITIONS-4

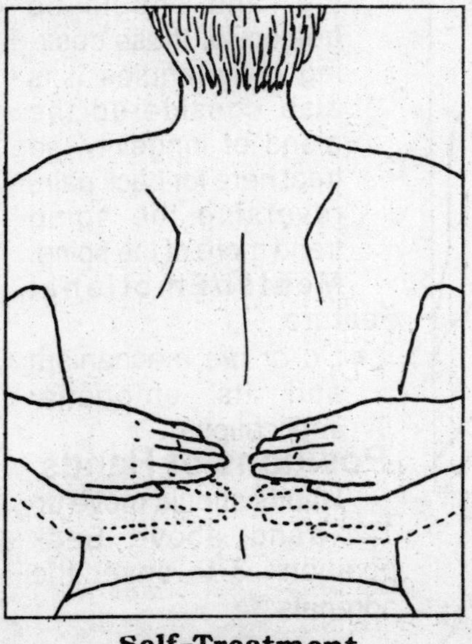

**Self-Treatment**

**POINTS TO REMEMBER**

Whenever one feels excitement the adrenal glands pump adrenalin throughout body and then we have situations of either adrenalin overload, where the body has more adrenalin than it needs on a regular basis, or adrenal failure, where it is used too much and breaks down.

Now the adrenal addiction should be dealt with strictness, because the people become addicted to the adrenalin rush.

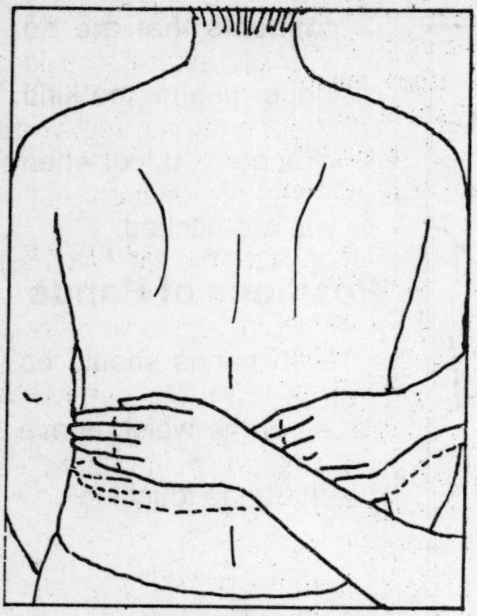

Person on chair

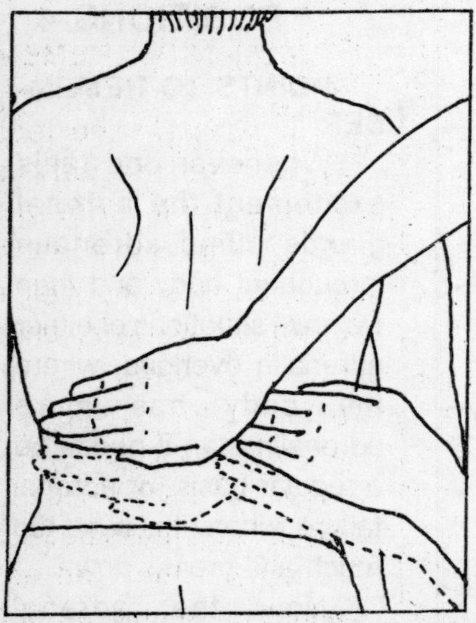

Person on table

**The Chakra**

Back of solar plexus *(see Front 2 & 3)*

**Oriental Faith**

This basically treats the kidneys. This is where the essential spark of our genetic potential is lit at conception. As the embryo develops, it unfolds from this area. As such, this area relates to one's destiny. This position balances willfulness. Destiny is arrived at when one aligns the personal will with the will of God.

**Physical Features**

- For immune system disorder—EBV, CFS, HIV+, AIDS, cancer, environmental allergies, etc. In Oriental medicine, this is the door of life, and should be treated for those desiring pregnancies it is also considered the gland of longevity, so treat here for back pain, reversing the aging trend more of the spine.

**Mental/Emotional Feature**

- *Do or die* mechanism and its emotional implications.

## Positions of Hands

Hands should move up 1/2 hand above Back position—3 to cover the adrenals

# BACK * * * * * * * * * * *POSITIONS-5&6

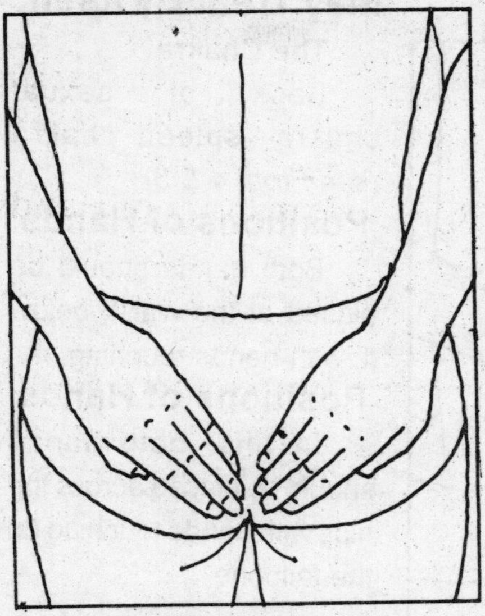

**Self-Treatment**

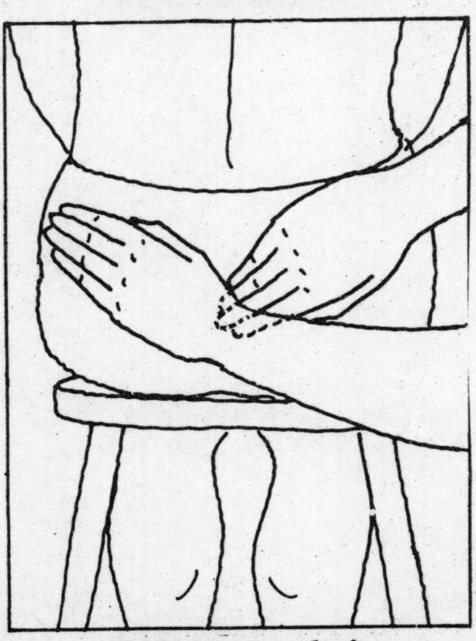

**Person on chair**

5 & 6 together are able to treat:

**Physical**

- Sciatic nerve problems
- lower back pain
- back of small and large intestines
- back of colon
- more of spine

**Chakra**

- root
- sexual
- spleen

## BACK—5

## May Treat By Itself:

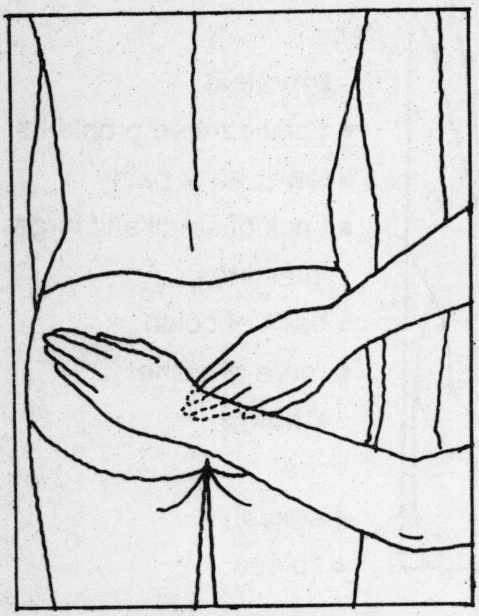

Person on table

**The Chakra**

Back of sexual chakra—spleen chakra *(see Front 4 & 5)*

### Positions of Hands

Both hands should be placed at the waist, below it, with hands touching.

### Positions of Hands

In this, both hands should be placed across the hips with hands touching on the tailbone

# REIKI FINISH

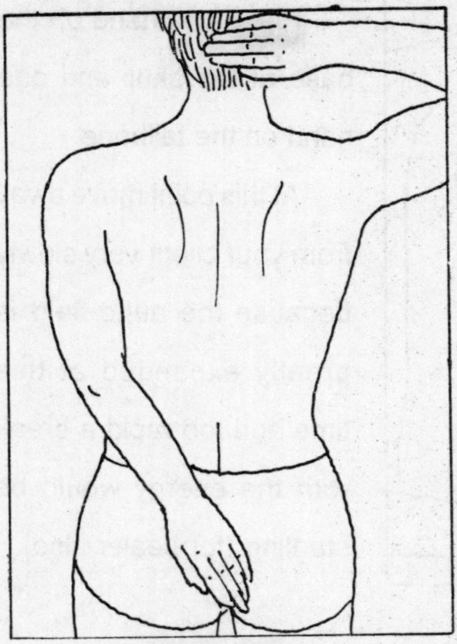

**Self-Treatment**

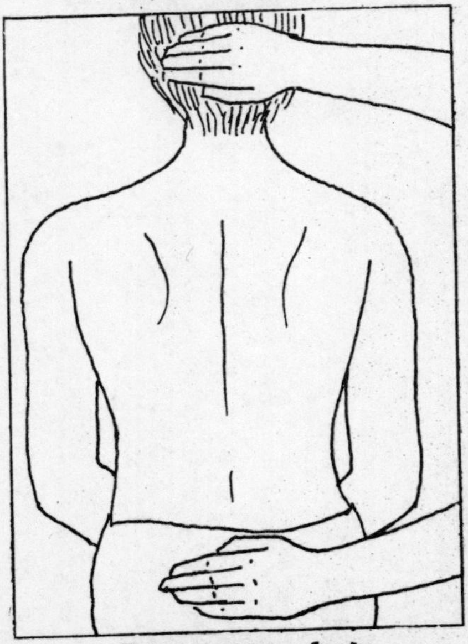

**Person on chair**

**Oriental Faith**

Their is a para sympathetic nerve plexus at the tailbone. Treating this area with the base of the neck amplifies para sympathetic resonance within the system. This adds the vitalizing healing properties of Reiki to the biological connections of the nervous system, creating a deeply relaxed field of energy. This is a powerful combination and its healing power should not be underestimated.

This position runs energy up and down the spine, and gives a very effective and soothing finish to the Reiki treatment.

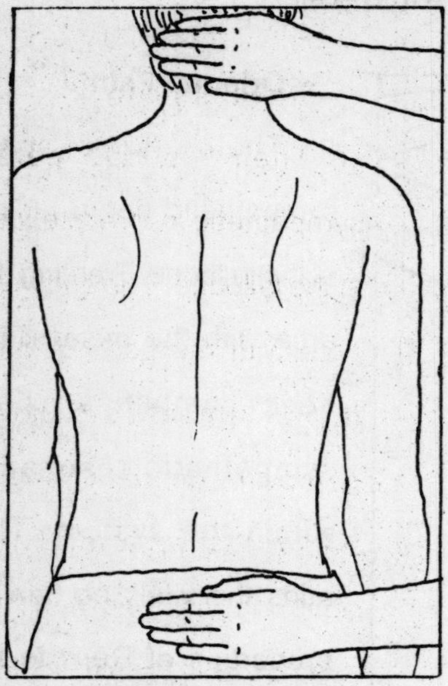

Person on table

## Positions of Hands

Place one hand on the base of the skull and one hand on the tailbone.

At this point move away from your client very slowly because the auric field is greatly expanded at this time and too rapid a break with the energy would be startling (for healer also).

# TREATMENT OF SPECIFIC DISORDERS

The disorders fall under two categories— acute and chronic disease. Acute problems are of a short duration, and usually react in a different way to Reiki treatments than chronic problems which have a longer duration. The major difference between the two categories is that acute cases usually involve an immediate healing crisis whereas chronic cases experience a healing crisis much later or not at all during the course of Reiki treatment.

Before starting any specific treatment, give a full treatment by applying all hand positions given in preceding section, then spend additional time on the positions listed. Repeat this pattern daily for three days to start the healing process, and then as needed. This is the best way to give a treatment though many times you will not have the time to do a full treatment, hence, do that whenever it is possible.

Five minutes spent on every position is appropriate time to help someone in good health advance to optimal health, you cannot do too much or too little Reiki, sometimes many hours of Reiki may be needed to facilitate a balance of the energy in a problem area. Typical problem like fractures, etc., require many hours "in person" and "absentee" treatments daily.

If a client with a chronic problem, such as backache, begins a series of Reiki treaments, the pain usually dissipates rapidly during the first few sessions. If the treatments are given over a period of several weeks, the pain and restlessness generally continue to disappear until the disease reaches the point of physical chemicalization. It is at this stage that the client may experience a relapse, and feel the effects of the complication even more painfully than before the beginning of treatment. This is a sign that you have reached the final level of toxic build-up, where the last vestiges of the disease are entrenched. As the Reiki energy makes contact with this final layer of toxins, the reaction resembles the last flicker of candle-stick. Likewise, the powerful energy of Reiki, purges disease with a strong current of Life Force Energy.

Do not forget to explain this to your client that physical chemicalization is an unpleasant but favourable symptom, hence, he should not discontinue treatments until the healing crisis has passed. It should be noted that occasionally a healing crisis does not occur and the symptom may just dwindle as the layers of toxins slowly pass away. Therefore, in chronic cases it is appropriate not to mention beforehand the possibility of physical chemicalization as it may never arise in a noticeable manner. Thus, it is better to wait, and if it does occur you can assure the patient that it is a positive sign, so he should not take it otherwise.

The acute cases are totally different. Generally, the person is in pain, as the disease is relatively new. If the patient has already visited a doctor, then your function is only to speed up the healing process. If not, and the situation is extremely critical, it is best to refer him to a qualified physician. When treating an acute problem, Reiki treatments often tend to initially intensify the pain, because a large amount of healing energy drawn to the problem area creates a sense of pressure. This symptom usually dissipates within two to three days, and relief of the problem is usually very rapid. It does not mean that it happens in Reiki treatment only, the acute symptoms react this way to many different methods of healing also.

In most of the spiritual and psychic healing methods, it takes a lag of few days for healings on the etheric body to finally affect the physical body. With Reiki there is no such kind of time required, because it is focused into both the physical and etheric bodies during treatment. As the healee draws the energy in, he/she also determines the length of treatment required.

Hence, whenever the healer is dealing with an acute healing problem, it is wise to inform the person that they might experience more discomfort for the first couple of days, until the symptoms begin to dissipate. Unlike dealing with chronic problems, which may or may not manifest a healing crisis, acute cases seem to produce more intense symptoms during the initial healing phase. Hence, it is wise to have the person prepared by properly informing them of the common reactions to such cases, so that this though may not nag them that their problem is getting worse.

Sometimes healers receive a complaint of pain or discomfort from a person who has been treated and was not suffering from any ailment beforehand. People sometimes have diseases or illnesses building up in their bodies, and are totally unaware of it. Reiki treatments can accelerate the healing energy in that area, which in turn, may be experienced as pain or discomfort, and it confuses a client.

Reiki speeds up the healing process of the body in a surprising manner. Suppose there is an infected cut on the skin. As the white blood cells rush to the infection and devour all of the invading bacteria, the feeling of pressure from all of the healing activity may cause pain.

It should be kept in mind that the unpleasant physical symptoms often are only signs that the body is operating properly in accomplishing all of the tasks needed to complete the healing process, so those symptoms should not be considered as indications of worsening condition.

This point should also be kept in mind that Reiki can penetrate any solid matter, such as cloth, wood, or steel. Reiki can also penetrate a plaster cast, while treating a broken bone. It is wise to wait until after a bone is properly set to treat it directly. If you need to treat a person who feels uncomfortable with having someone touch them physically, you can transmit Reiki by allowing your hands to hover just above the body. Reiki treatments are highly recommended for patients who are going to have surgery. It is best to treat them only before and after the operation, because Reiki can speed up the effect of the anesthesia on the body and cause it to wear off prematurely. Never do Reiki treatment during surgery.

Hawayo Takata taught a simple pattern of hand positions which follow the endocrine system. She often added a few of her own positions as other Reiki Masters have done. You can use them for self-treatments or for working on others:

Start treatment by placing palms over your eyes. Other areas of the body can be included as well. Use your intuition as guide as to what is appropriate. Whenever there is a specific disorder, such as diabetes, you should treat the appropriate internal organs that are affected by the disease, which, in this case, would be the pancreas. If there is a liver problem, of course you would focus on the liver. Also, it is good to spend at least thirty minutes per day on the specific disease areas of the body, such as a malignant tumour in the case of cancer. Try to spend time on the endocrine system and place special emphasis on the thymus gland, which has a powerful effect on the immune system. Use your intuition to guide you, and keep your hands on areas which continue to draw energy, for as long as possible. Signals which tell you when it is time to change position are varied. You will come to know when the patient will take a deep sigh of relief, feel the heat begin to decrease in your hands, or feel the pulsations or tingling subside. The intuitive sense that it's time to change positions is quite adequate. The average time to spend in each area is approximately three to five minutes, but can be extended as required.

Remember that when treating any person, no matter how emotionally bonded the healer may be, he must not have any attachments to the consequences of his healing.

This is the most difficult task for a healer to let go and allow each person to decide whether they want to get well or stay sick, to live or to die peacefully.

Helping someone with Reiki during the process of dying is a very spiritual experience. The birth and death are both transitions. The love energy inherent in each experience is so overwhelming that the true feeling cannot be expressed in words. The essential factor in each is that one is dealing with the whole perfect person in the true sense of the word. Babies are born as perfect whole beings, and during the death process all of the old dross is shed, revealing the true beauty of the person in transition.

Reiki gives you two options "self-treatment" and treating others. Some situations are best treated as "self-treatments" because of the many hours of treatment needed. Other treatments are best done by another person because of the difficulty in reaching certain areas of the body or because of the weak state of the sufferer. It is always recommended that people should also learn Reiki to treat themselves between their sessions with a practitioner, it will prove to be highly beneficial.

Most miraculous results can be observed while treating infants, accidents and animals: infants because they grow pretty quickly;. accidents because the injury seldom has a chance to get into cellular memory; and animals, because they are naturally open to receive Life Force Energy.

The healer should also look for the metaphysical causes for the disease. Most illness have metaphysical causes, and that only when we start working to heal the metaphysical causes we achieve desired results within a short span of time.

It is recommended to those who are suffering from some chronic problems that they, and all their close family members, should learn both First and Second Degree Reiki.

The healer must use common sense and seek whatever professional help may be needed, both with accidents and with chronic problems, because Reiki is not meant to be replaced with appropriate medical care.

# REIKI TREATMENTS

**ABSCESS**—The abscess should be covered with a tissue and treated for 30 minutes, (preferably twice daily), then the spleen should be treated to help cleanse and purify the blood. The abscess should be treated till it breaks or is reabsorbed by the body.

**ACCIDENTS**—The injured area should be treated directly (especially if there is profuse bleeding) and treat on the adrenals, BACK 4, and over the solar plexus, FRONT 2 & 3. Get appropriate medical help immediately if it is required.

**ACNE**—The affected area should be treated directly and also apply HEAD 3, treat the spleen for blood purification, FRONT 4 & 5, and BACK 5 & 6 to help release toxins from the body faster. Frequently a colon cleanse program, when used in addition to Reiki treatments, will help to speed the healing process. Treatment for allergies should also be given.

**ACUPRESSURE**—*See* **ACUPUNCTURE.**

**ACUPUNCTURE**—If an acupuncturist had Reiki, the Reiki energy flows through the acupuncturist's hands, directly into, and through, the needles into the acupuncture point. In such condition releases tend to be quicker and longer lasting.

**ADDICTIONS**—There should be an eclectic approach in treating any addiction, and Reiki should be an integral part of a program that includes abstinence, a Twelve Step Program (AA, OA, NA, etc.), counseling, vitamin and mineral therapy, and detoxing. Treat HEAD 3 for the old brain, FRONT 2 & 3 for the liver, FRONT 4 & 5, and BACK 5 & 6 for the release of toxins, and BACK 4 for the adrenals.

**ADRENALS**—Adrenalin depletion as well as adrenal overload or failure are all common today. Treat on the adrenals, BACK 4, for as long and as often as possible, but a minimum of 30 minutes a day. Changes in lifestyle are also essential to overcome this complication.

**AGING**—Reiki appears to slow down the aging process when used in conjunction with a healthy lifestyle (vitamin and mineral intakes, exercise, mental attitude, diet, etc.). Reiki reverses the aging process by reversing the increase in entropy.

It does this directly, and also indirectly by rebalancing the subtle bodies and chakras.

Besides a daily full body treatment, treat HEAD 1, 2, 3, and FRONT 1. In addition, treat any areas that are causing discomfort or existing problems.

**AIDS**—*See* **IMMUNE SYSTEM DISORDERS.**

**ALLERGIES**—First of all take care of the cause of the allergy from the diet, or from the environment. Many people have unrecognized allergies to some vegetables, dairy products, wheat products, food additives, white sugar, red meat and lentils. In the environment, some major troublemakers are fume, dust, dog and cat fluff of, mattress mites, and smell of fabric and paints Balls of fluff and dust of carpet, etc. Treat HEAD 1 & 3 to clear the sinuses and to treat the old brain, FRONT 1 for the lungs, 2 & 3 for the digestion, 4 & 5 for detoxing, and at least 30 minutes daily on BACK 4 for the adrenals.

**AMYOTROPHIC LATERAL SCLEROSIS**—Full hands on treatment, with 2nd Degree. At least twice daily with additional time on HEAD 1 2 & 3, FRONT 1, and from top to bottom of the spine.

**ALZHEIMER'S**—Full hands-on treatment, with 2nd Degree, twice daily with extra time on HEAD 1 2 & 3.

**ANEMIA**—Treat the spleen (left side above the waist), and the adrenals, BACK 4. **ANOREXIA** *See* **ADDICTIONS.**

**ANXIETY**—Apply HEAD 1 2 & 3 to bring emotional balance, FRONT 2 & 3 for centering and BACK 4 for the adrenals.

**ARMS, LEGS, HANDS AND FEET**—Treat any joint or muscle problem directly on the area of need, sandwiching it between hands.

**ARTHRITIS**—*See* **AUTO-IMMUNE SYSTEM DISORDERS.**

**ASTHMA**—*See* **ALLERGIES.** Second Degree hands are essentially required for the treatments. After the full body treatment, also add 30 minutes of treatments on each side of the pleura, the side of the lungs, by placing both hands on the side of the torso above the waist while the person is lying on their opposite side. Treat for 21 consecutive days without a break in number of days.

**AUTO—IMMUNE SYSTEM DISORDERS (Arthritis, Pernicious Anaemia etc.)**—It is essential to take a close look at one's diet every now and then. Many arthritic type problems are helped by eliminating certain foods that are toxic to the sufferer. Many people also get relief from treatments and herbal supplements given by an Oriental Medical Doctor/Licensed Acupuncturist. Apply HEAD 3 for the old brain, FRONT 5 for the bladder, BACK 3 for the kidneys, and BACK 4 for the adrenals. Spend additional time on any painful or swollen areas to break up the calcium deposits. To flush toxins from the system the intake of liquids should be appropriate.

**BACKACHES**—In condition of acute pain, treat directly on the problem area. For chronic pain, start at the base of the skull and treat all of the way down the spine to the tail bone. Also give additional time to FRONT 5 & 6. The metaphysical cause of the condition should also be considered and treated accordingly.

**BALDNESS**—Direct treatment over the bald spots daily and for as long as possible is recommended. This is best done by another person since many hours of treatment are required. However, Reiki treatment had been known to regenerate hair growth for many people. Massage vitamin E oil into the scalp each evening, and shampoo the head each morning with some nourishing shampoo.

**BED WETTING**—Apply FRONT 5 & BACK 6 to strengthen the bladder.

**BEE STINGS**—First of all, remove the stinger if possible. Gently suck on the wound for about a minute, spitting out the venom frequently (it should not be done if you have any type of sore in your mouth or on your lips). Place one hand on the wound and the other either above the wound (toward the heart), or on the opposite side if the wound is on an arm or leg. Treat for at least 20 to 30 minutes. If the person's condition is critical then also treat the lymphatic system, both sides of the neck, thymus area, groin and under the arms.

**BLEEDING**—The wound should be covered with a clean cloth and treated directly if possible. If you are concerned about exposure to the blood then cover the cloth with a plastic covering.

**BLISTERS**—*See* **BURNS.**

**BLOOD PRESSURE**—Both high and low blood pressure

can be balanced by treating HEAD 3 & 4, and FRONT 1. Yogic breathing, guided visualizations, and biofeedback are also extremely helpful in these problems.

**BOILS**—*See* **ABSCESS.**

**BRAIN INJURY** or **TUMOURS**—Give as much time as possible on all 4 head positions, and add hand positions on each side of the head, if required. Remember that with head injuries there is often damage on the side of the head opposite the injury.

**BREASTS**—For any kind of breast problem (male or female), cancer, abscesses, lumps, etc., treatment should be done directly on the breast area. Unless the person is your partner it is illegal to give such a treatment. It is therefore recommended that the person should have Reiki for herself. The treatment consists of as much time as possible directly on the breasts, and at least 20 minutes on FRONT 5.

**BROKEN BONES**—Never treat directly on the break until after it has been set. Instead treat above and below the break. As soon as the break has been set, treat through the cast for as many hours as possible, with Second Degree.

**BRONCHITIS**—*See* **ALLERGIES.**

**BULIMIA**—*See* **ADDICTIONS.**

**BURNS**—Place hands directly over, but never on the burnt area. Treat for 15 minutes or until after the pain goes away, then apply BACK 4 for the adrenals.

**BURSITIS**—*See* **ARTHRITIS.**

**CALLUSES CORNS**—Ask the person to go for a Chiropractic checkup of the spine, legs and feet. Treat the spine, hips, and the area of the foot that is involved.

**CANCER**—*See* **IMMUNE SYSTEM DISORDERS.**

**CARBUNCLE**—*See* **ABSCESS.**

**CATARACT**—*See* **EYES.**

**CEREBRAL PALSY**—Daily treatments are essential with additional time spent on treating HEAD 2 & 3, FRONT 1 2 & 3, and BACK 3.

**CHEMOTHERAPY**—Full 2nd Degree treatments daily with additional time on spleen, liver and adrenals.

**CHILDBIRTH**—Give treatment as much as possible during the pregnancy giving the mother full treatments and covering the entire abdominal area. During labour, have as many people as possible doing absentee treatments on both mother and child. Treat the mother hands-on during the labour process on BACK 5 & 6, the lower back, and the total abdominal area, FRONT 3 down through 5 with as many added hand positions as required.

**CHRONIC FATIGUE SYNDROME**—*See* **IMMUNE SYSTEM DISORDER.**

**CIRRHOSIS OF THE LIVER**—*See* **LIVER.**

**CIRCULATION**—Start treatment with HEAD 3 and 4, then FRONT 1 and 5. If you are treating yourself or your partner, you may also treat the groin area by placing the middle finger of one hand on the large artery going to the leg (the soft spot just behind the tendon that goes from the torso down into the leg), and the other hand on FRONT 4. Circulation in the hands is improved by having Reiki for yourself and running the energy through them by giving various treatments.

**COLDS**—Give treatment twice daily for 3 consecutive days giving a full treatment each time, then extra time on FRONT 1 & 5. In addition, for head colds spend additional time on HEAD 1, 2 & 3, and for chest colds spend additional time on HEAD 4, FRONT 2, BACK 1 & 2 and on both sides of the rib cage.

**COLIC**—Hold the baby in such a manner that one hand treats the stomach area and the other hand treats the back. Treat until gas is released and the baby is relieved of discomfort. A very extended treatment has been known to clear up the problem in some cases.

**COMA**—Spend additional time on HEAD 1 2 & 3, on FRONT 1 2 & 3, and on BACK 4. Group treatments are especially helpful and absentee treatments are also effective in such cases.

**COMPULSIVE OVEREATING**—*See* **OBESITY** and **ADDICTIONS.**

**CONGENITAL DEFECTS**—The birth defects should be treated in the womb if possible and require full body treatments as quickly after birth as possible. The problem is rarely cured, but improvements have occurred when treatment was begun early in the pregnancy. It is also helpful for the child to have First Degree so that whenever they touch themselves they run the energy.

**CONSTIPATION**—Apply HEAD 3, FRONT 4 & 5, and BACK 5 & 6.

**COUGHS**—*See* **COLDS.** Spend additional time on the diaphragm, FRONT 2.

**CRAMPS**—*See* **MENSTRUAL PROBLEMS.**

**CUTS**—Give immediate treatment to stop the bleeding and to seal the cut. Clean the wound, bandage and continue to treat. Call for medical care if stitches are necessary and continue treating as much as possible to speed up the healing process.

**CYSTIC FIBROSIS**—Full treatments daily with additional time on HEAD 3, FRONT 1 & 2, BACK 1 & 2 and both pleuras.

**CYSTITIS**—Apply FRONT 5, BACK 6 and spleen.

**CYSTS**—*See* **ABSCESS.**

**DEAFNESS**—*See* **EARS.**

**DENTAL PROBLEMS**—Give direct treatment on the problem area (directly in the mouth if doing self-treatment).

**DEPRESSION**—*See* **EMOTIONAL DISORDERS.**

**DETACHED RETINA**—Spend additional time on HEAD 1. Also treat HEAD 2 & 3.

**DIABETES**—If the person is on insulin, make sure that he keeps very close watch on his insulin needs since there will usually be a dramatic drop in insulin requirements. Apply HEAD 3, FRONT 2 (minimum of 30 minutes) & 3, and BACK 4. If there is a problem, or a potential problem, with diabetic blindness treat HEAD 1, 2, 3, and FRONT 5 for women (ovaries), or BACK 6 for men (prostate).

**DIALYSIS**—Reiki should be used to lessen the cramping while on a dialysis machine by treating directly on the muscles involved. Daily Second Degree treatments are needed with additional time spent on the liver, spleen, FRONT 4 & 5, and BACK 3, 5, & 6.

**DIARRHOEA**—Treat on FRONT 4 & 5, and BACK 5 & 6.

**DIGESTIVE DISORDERS**—Start treatment with HEAD 3 then proceed to FRONT 2 & 3, FRONT 4 & 5, and BACK 5 & 6.

**DIVERTICULOSIS**—*See* **DIARRHOEA.**

**DIZZINESS**—*See* **EQUILIBRIUM PROBLEMS.**

**DROPPED FOOT**—This particular hand position can be used only on your partner for legal reasons. Ask your partner to lie on the back with legs spread apart, knees bent slightly. Then place your middle finger on the groin area where the leg joins the body, and the other hand on FRONT 5 on the same side of the body. Proceed to treat the foot, the ankle and the calf by sandwiching each area between your hands.

**DRUG ADDICTION**—*See* **ADDICTIONS.**

**EARS**—Place the middle fingers gently and directly into the ear and the other fingers close in, both in front of the ears and behind them. If the ear is too tender for the fingers to be placed in then cup the hands over the ears. This method is less direct and will take longer time.

**EDEMA**—Fluid retention can be relieved by treating HEAD 3, FRONT 4 & 5, and BACK 3 & 4. Take some medicine which may help increase the excretion of urine.

**EMOTIONAL DISORDERS**—In this complication HEAD 2 is the primary treatment position. It is beneficial to also give additional time to HEAD 1 & 3, FRONT 2 & 3, and BACK 4. Use of the Second Degree Mental, Emotional and Addictive treatment is also highly beneficial.

**EMPHYSEMA**—*See* **ALLERGIES.** In this regular treatment is necessary for 30 consecutive days. If treatment is discontinued before the total 30 days, then you must start back at Day number 1 of the treatment series.

**ENERGIZING**—Place one hand on the navel and the other on the Solar Plexus.

**EPILEPSY**—Apply HEAD 2. Start the treatment at the onset of the seizure, and continue for as long as possible.

**EQUILIBRIUM PROBLEMS**—HEAD 2 should be the primary position, also treat HEAD 1 & 3, and both ears.

**EYES**—Apply HEAD 1 2 & 3 so that both eyes and eye stems are completely treated. Frequently there are also related glandular problems in need of treatment. This is the treatment for cataracts, near-sightedness or far-sightedness, infections and glaucoma.

**FASTING**—Treatments twice in a day will help replenish your vital life force energy and speed up the cleansing process. Spend additional time on HEAD 3, FRONT 4 & 5, and BACK 3, 5 & 6.

**FATIGUE**—Apply HEAD 1 & 3, FRONT 3, and BACK 4.

Sleeping with one or both hands as in HEAD 3 will quicken the balancing process.

**FEET**—*See* **ARMS.**

**FEVER**—Fevers can usually be broken with a full treatment and extra time on HEAD 3 & 4, and BACK 4.

**FIBROMYALGIA SYNDROME**—Give full treatments daily, and recommend a hand on HEAD 3 for going to sleep. Spend extra time on knees, elbows, upper thigh on the back of the leg, and on the spleen.

**FLU**—*See* **COLDS.**

**FOOD POISONING**—Spend additional time on FRONT 2, 3, 4, & 5, and on BACK 3, 5 & 6.

**FRACTURES**—*See* **BROKEN BONES.**

**FROSTBITE**—Treat at once on the affected areas and on BACK 4 for the adrenals. Then give a full body treatment immediately.

**GALL BLADDER**—Treat the right side of both FRONT 2 & 3, and the right side of BACK 4. Frequently a "glug-glug" sound will be both heard and felt when giving direct treatment over the gall bladder as it releases.

**GALLSTONES**—*See* **GALL BLADDER**. A long treatment or several shorter treatments will frequently pulverize the stones so they may be expelled.

**GAS**—*See* **DIARRHOEA.**

**GLAUCOMA**—*See* **EYES.**

**GOUT**—*See* **ARTHRITIS.** Also eat cherries or drink cherry juice.

**GROUNDING**—Firmly hold soles of the feet, then place one hand on the Solar Plexus and the other on the navel, or place one hand on the top of the head and the other on the Solar Plexus.

**HAIR**—*See* **BALDNESS.**

**HANDS**—*See* **ARMS.**

**HANGOVER**—Apply Head 1, 2 & 3, FRONT 2 & 3, and BACK 4.

**HEAD INJURIES**—*See* **BRAIN INJURIES.**

**HEADACHE (Migraine)**—Apply FRONT 1, 2, 3, & 4, then 30 minutes on FRONT 5 for women, or BACK 6 for men, since there appears to be a link between migraines and ovaries or prostate. Next treat HEAD 1, 2 & 3. Treatment of minimum three consecutive days is required.

**HEADACHE (Caused by Tension)**—Apply HEAD 1, 2, 3 & 4, FRONT 2 & 3 to detox the liver, Front 5 & 6 to speed up the release of toxins, and BACK 1 for shoulder tension. Try to remove the cause of the tension and do a neck and shoulder release. Chiropractic adjustments are frequently called for and regular massages can help to keep the body's tension level down. For stress reduction and replacing the vitamins depleted by stress take Vitamin B Complex.

**HEART ATTACK**—Call for professional help at once. Then place both hands over the heart/diaphragm area (at centre on left side of the body). After that you can progress to FRONT 1, 2 and BACK 4 for the adrenals.

**HEARTBURN**—Apply HEAD 3, FRONT 2 & 3.

**HEMATOMA**—First of all, give full body treatment, then place hands directly over the swollen area. Blood is re-absorbed by the body.

**HEMOPHILIA**—Apply HEAD 3 for the old brain, and FRONT 2 & 3 for pancreas.

**HAEMORRHAGE**—Call for professional help at once. Place one hand over the problem area and the other over the heart. It is always best to protect yourself with latex so the direct exposure to someone else's blood can be avoided.

**HAEMORRHOIDS**—This complication should be treated with a variation of BACK 6: put the middle finger directly over the anal opening, and the other hand across the base of the spine. Treat for 30 minutes. (For legal reasons this treatment must only be done on yourself or your partner.)

**HEPATITIS**—*See* **LIVER.**

**HERNIA**—Direct treatment on the hernia—after the projection has been placed back into the opening, is recommended.

**HERNIA (Hiatal)** Direct treatment over the diaphragm, FRONT 2 is recommended. An old treatment used with Reiki is to drink a glass of water, hold your hands above your head, and jump up and down several times, this is an effective treatment.

**HERPES**—Treatment to reduce stress and direct treatment on the affected area for as long as possible is recommended.

**HICCUPS**—Instruct the sufferer to lie down with his arms stretched over his head. Place one hand on the base of the breast bone, and the other directly below it. For self-treatment, place both hands in this same position, one hand above and the other on the breast bone. Treat until the hiccups vanish.

**HIGH BLOOD PRESSURE**—Start the treatment with HEAD 4 to treat the carotid arteries, but do not forget to treat the old brain, Head 3 also. Guided visualizaion and biofeedback are excellent modalities for lowering blood pressure. Be careful about your diet.

**HIV POSITIVE**—*See* **IMMUNE SYSTEM DISORDERS.**

**HYPERTENSION**—*See* **HIGH BLOOD PRESSURE.**

**HYPOGLYCEMIA**—Full treatments daily with additional time on HEAD 3, FRONT 2 (minimum of 30 minutes), and 3, and BACK 4.

**IMMUNE SYSTEM DISORDERS**—Lupus, Chronic Fatigue Syndrome (CFS), Epstein-Barr Virus (EBV), HIV+, AIDS, Cancer, Crohn's Disease etc. This treatment covers any breakdown of the immune system. Treat HEAD POSITIONS 2, 3 & 4, FRONT 1 & 5, BACK 4, spleen, and any particular area involved.

**IMPOTENCE**—Apply HEAD 3, FRONT 5, BACK 4 & 6 for the adrenals. Treat directly over the prostate if you are treating yourself or your partner.

**INDIGESTION**—*See* **DIGESTIVE DISORDERS.**

**INFECTIONS**—Apply HEAD 3, BACK 4, on the left side for the spleen, and directly on the infection.

**INFLUENZA**—*See* **COLDS.**

**INSECT BITES**—*See* **BEE STINGS.**

**INSOMNIA**—*See* **SLEEP DISORDERS.**

**JAUNDICE**—*See* **LIVER.**

**LARYNGITIS**—Give direct treatment on the throat. Look for the metaphysical cause, it might be due to something said, inability to speak up for oneself, check on expressing oneself, etc.

**LEARNING AND MEMORY**—The initial position is HEAD 2, however, time should also be given on HEAD 3 & 4 and from 3. It has also been observed that quiet peaceful music can also be of great help.

**LEGS**—*See* **ARMS.**

**LIVER**—For completely covering the liver, which is on the right side of the body, start treatment with both hands, one above the other, to the right of the front centre line of the body. Continue working your way around the body until you reach the centre of the back. This is a time consuming treatment and is in addition to, not instead of, a full treatment.

**MASSAGE**—Start a massage by applying Reiki for 5 minutes on HEAD 1 or 2 to tap into the energy. Continue by doing your usual massage, then end the massage. Spending 5 minutes on the soles of the feet. Reiki can be used to enhance any massage modality.

**MEASLES**—Give a body treatment immediately to adults but wait 24 hours before treating children. Spend additional time on HEAD 1.

**MEMORY**—*See* **LEARNING & MEMORY.**

**MENOPAUSE**—Apply HEAD 3 for the old brain, FRONT 2 & 3 on the right side for the liver, FRONT 5 for the ovaries, BACK 4 for the adrenals, and BACK 6 for the back of the ovaries. In the East there are many miraculous herbs to help with menopause and acupuncture needles can also release many blockages that cause problems.

**MENSTRUAL PROBLEMS**—Start treatment 4 to 5 days before the onset of menses and continue throughout the period. Apply HEAD 3, FRONT 5, and BACK 6. Frequently, taking calcium-magnesium supplements and a herbal diuretic will help alleviate the pain.

**MIGRAINE**—*See* **HEADACHE.**

**MOLES & WARTS**—These can be treated effectively by pinching gently between the fingers as often as possible and they will usually dry up and drop off.

**MOTION SICKNESS**—The primary treatment areas of this inner ear problem, are HEAD 2, 3, and 4, along with FRONT 2.

**MOUTH SORES**—*See* **DENTAL PROBLEMS.**

**MULTIPLE SCLEROSIS**—Give full Second Degree treatments twice daily, with additional time on HEAD 2 & 3, FRONT 2 & 3, and on the spine from top to bottom, and end with the Reiki Finish. The client should be taught Reiki and asked to keep their hands on themselves whenever it is possible.

**MUMPS**—Give a full body treatment immediately to adults but wait 24 hours before treating a child. Additional time should be spent on the spleen and areas of concentration of lymph glands (grain, underarms and throat), with 30 spent treating the ovaries or testicles (only on yourself or your partner for legal reasons).

**MUSCULAR DYSTROPHY**—Give full Second Degree treatments twice daily with additional time on HEAD 1, 2, & 3, FRONT 1, 2, & 3, and BACK 2 & 3. The client should be taught Reiki and asked to keep their hands on themselves whenever it is possible for them.

**NAUSEA**—Apply HEAD 3, FRONT 2 & 3. Vomiting is possible since the body sometimes detoxes rapidly due to Reiki.

**NERVOUSNESS**—*See* **EMOTIONAL DISORDERS.**

**NOSEBLEED**—The sufferer should be placed at a 45 degree angle with an ice bag on the backside of the neck. Cup hand around the nose with thumb on one side and fingers balled up on the other to block the nasal opening. Place other hand on the base of the skull.

**OBESITY**—*See* **ADDICTIONS**— Besides this apply HEAD 3 for old brain & 4 for thyroid, FRONT 2 & 3 for liver and digestion, and FRONT 4 & 5 for detoxing. A regular colon cleanse is helpful. The eating habits should also be changed for weight reduction.

**PAIN**—You will find a soft spot on the top of the shoulders next to the bone, that is a major endorphin-releasing spot for the body. Treat this spot for pain anywhere in the body because endorphins are a natural morphine the body produces. Please note that morphine is administered in the patients who suffer from extremely painful conditions.

**PARALYSIS**—Give full body treatments twice daily, additional time on HEAD 3, BACK 4, and on the affected areas is recommended. The client should be taught Reiki and asked to keep their hands on themselves whenever possible, and to do full body treatments with the Second Degree Absentee technique several times in a day.

**PARKINSON'S DISEASE**—Full treatments twice daily are essential with additional time spent on HEAD 1, 2, 3, and 4, FRONT 2, BACK 4, and both hands.

**PLEURISY**—*See* **COLDS.**

**PNEUMONIA**—Do the whole treatment with client lying on his back with head and upper torso slightly elevated. Spend additional time on HEAD 1, 2, 3, & 4, FRONT 1, 2, & 3, top on the shoulders, and by slipping the hands under the body apply BACK 2 & 4. In non-critical conditions treat daily until the fever breaks (usually 4 or 5 days). In critical situations treat continuously if possible until the fever breaks (could take 4 to 5 hours). Team and absentee treatments are also highly recommended wherever possible.

**PROSTATE**—The direct treatment on the prostate gland is recommended primarily. This can only be done on yourself or your partner for legal reasons. Also apply HEAD 4 for the thyroid gland.

**PSORIASIS**—Full treatments (daily) with additional time on HEAD 3 and directly on the scaley areas is recommended.

**PYORRHOEA**—*See* **DENTAL & GUM PROBLEMS.** On 10 consecutive days treat for 30 minutes on the mouth and 10 minutes on the spleen besides full body treatment.

**RADIATION**—Full treatments with extra time on the spleen and on the area exposed to the radiation are recommended twice daily. Epsom salts baths also help a lot to draw out the toxins or waste products.

**RASH**—Direct treatment on the problem area is recommended. Check for allergies or other possible causes. A change of diet may also be required.

**REFLEXOLOGY**—Reiki reaches the reflex points directly and facilitates quick releases that last longer than they do without Reiki.

**RINGING IN THE EARS**—*See* **EARS**

**SCARS**—Give direct treatment over the scar tissue as regularly and as long as possible. Very little can be expected if the scar is over 2 years old. Fasting is considered by some to help dissolve scars.

**SCIATIC NERVE PROBLEMS**—Start treatment with the fingers of both hands touching the spine, with the upper hand touching, but below, the waist. Be sure that as you work your way down the hip and leg that you overlap hand positions and do not miss even a fraction of an inch of space. As you get to the lower part of the hip start angling out so that you will be treating the upper-outer quadrant of the leg. Work your way down the entire leg and end the treatment in the arch of the foot. Draw the energy out and away from the body when you complete the treatment. This treatment will take from 1 to 2 hours and it is extremely difficult do on yourself, but it has been found to be quite effective.

**SCLERODERMA**—Full body treatments with additional time over the hardening areas are recommended daily.

**SENILITY**—Spend additional time on HEAD 1, 2, & 3, FRONT 1 for the heart, and BACK 4 for the adrenals.

**SEXUAL COMPLICATIONS**—Give extra time on HEAD 3, FRONT 5 and BACK 6. Treat directly on the vaginal area or the prostate if giving self-treatment or working on your partner (if it is permitted). If there is some emotional problem then apply FRONT 1 for the heart.

**SEXUALLY TRANSMITTED DISEASES**—Besides giving full body treatments, additional time should be spent on the spleen, the lymph glands (throat, underarms and groin) and BACK 4 for adrenals, and if you are working on yourself or your partner then direct treatment on the sexual organs is recommended.

**SHINGLES**—After going through a full treatment, place one hand below the breastbone and the other on the left shoulder blade and treat for 10 to 15 minutes, then treat all affected areas. Due to extreme sensitivity it may be necessary to treat above the affected areas, instead of touching them.

**SHOCK**—Call for professional help at once. Leave out a full treatment. Go directly to HEAD 2 & 3, FRONT 3 for the solar plexus, and then BACK 4 for the adrenals.

**SICKLE-CELL ANAEMIA**—Full treatments with extra time on spleen, liver, heart, lungs, joints and the full length of the arms and legs are recommended daily. The persons will have to learn Reiki themselves because of the extensive treatments required in this complication.

**SINUS**—Apply HEAD 1, 2 & 3 to get all sinus cavities, then. FRONT 1, BACK 1 & 2. Investigation for allergies is also required.

**SLEEP DISORDERS**—Start with a short treatment of HEAD 2, then place one hand on HEAD 3 and the other one on the solar plexus. Support your arms with pillows and try to fall asleep with your hands in this position. A mental, emotional and addictive treatment with Second Degree is also highly beneficial.

**SMOKING**—*See* **ADDICTIONS.**

**SNAKEBITE**—Start with appropriate first aid by placing a tight wrap between the wound and the heart. Place one hand on the wound and the other over blood vessels between the wound and the heart. If there are more Reiki Therapists available then ask them to treat the entire lymphatic system, neck, underarms, and groin (if legal), and BACK 4 for the adrenals.

**SPRAIN**—Treat directly on the sprain at once after the injury and for as long as possible.

**STRESS REDUCTION**—Reiki is one of the best method for stress reduction. By giving oneself daily treatments one can overcome this complication quite easily.

**STROKE**—Call for professional help at once. Full treatments twice daily are recommended for a minimum of 4 days, with extra time spent on HEAD 2, 3 & 4 (at least 1 hour), FRONT 1, 2 & 3, and BACK 4. Treat arms and/or legs if they are affected due to this problem.

**SUNBURN**—*See* **BURNS.**

**SURGERY**—Give treatment for as many days as possible before the surgery. Treat the patient, the doctors and the nurses involved during the surgery with Second Degree Absentee Treatments, and treat extensively after the surgery, both absentee and in person.

**TACHYCARDIA**—Give direct treatment over the heart.

**TENDINITIS**—Direct treatment on the area for at least 30 minutes daily is recommended. Check to see what repetitive motion is being made with the arm or leg and work to change to a different movement.

**THYROID PROBLEMS**—The Master Gland-thyroid, must function properly for the proper function of the whole body. Because of the tie in between the thyroid and the adrenal glands it is necessary to apply both FRONT 4 and BACK 4.

**TONSILLITIS**—Apply HEAD 3 & 4, under the lower jaw for 15 to 20 minutes, and on the spleen.

**TMJ—(Tempero-Mandibular Joint Dysfunction)** Treatment on both sides of the head in front of the ears, and at the base of the skull is recommended.

**TRANSITION**—Reiki offers easy death or dying process for the people, in which those who are working professionally will be able to be supportive during the process. Treat over FRONT 1 for the heart, and the Second Degree Absentee for the person in transition, the care givers, and those affected to ease the last journey for all.

**TUMOURS**—Treat directly on area of the tumour, for as much time as possible, in addition to that, daily full body treatment is also recommended. Some people tape their hands over the tumour while sleeping to get hours of treatment and they had been tremendously benefitted by this.

**ULCERS**—Apply full Reiki treatments daily to lower the stress level, and treat directly over the painful area as often as possible and for as long a time as possible. And try to remove causes of stress from your life.

**VARICOSE VEINS**—*See* **CIRCULATION.** Some extra time should be spent directly on the problem creating veins.

**VENEREAL DISEASES**—*See* **SEXUALLY TRANSMITTED DISEASES.**

**VOMITTING** *See* **NAUSEA.**

**WHIPLASH**— Apply HEAD 1, 2, 3 & 4. Treat also on the sides and back of the neck for 30 minutes or some more time.

## REIKI RESEARCHES

### Biofeedback and Blood Pressure

This scientifically designed research was carried out by Reiki Master teacher, Penny Devine, as part of a research project at the Evergreen State College, in Olympia, Washington. In this study, Penny worked closely with experts in both biofeedback and health, to ensure the validity of the results. Devine used measurements of vital statistics, biofeedback data and self-report to secure her data. The purpose of this study was to scientifically prove the effect of Reiki on stress release response.

Data and Vital signs (blood pressure, rate of heartbeat respiration and temperature) were taken on Reiki students at the beginning and end of the first day of a Reiki class, at the end of the complete class, and one week after the class. Clients were tested with biofeedback before a treatment started and throughout the entire treatment. Anecdotal data was determined through use of "The Change Scales", a participant profile form, and a form for self-evaluation of experiences during the Reiki class. A control group that had no exposure to Reiki had also gone through the same kind of testing at corresponding times.

That test resulted in an immediate confirmation, by changes on the graphs, of the therapist's perceptions of energy fluctuations. An increase in energy flow was indicated by an increase in extremity temperature, which was followed by a levelling-off of temperature at the same time as the therapist felt a decrease in the energy flow. Biofeedback Relaxation Response readings showed that all but one of the participants met the muscle relation norm, while all but three participants met the "low relaxed norm:" Twelve out of seventeen surpassed this norm, experiencing even deeper relaxation in 14 minutes. The testing of vital signs showed a significant lowering of all four indicators (blood pressure, rate of heartbeat respiration and temperature etc. of health.

This way Penny succeeded in her purpose of documenting positive effects of both Reiki treatments and Reiki training on stress/relaxation levels—in participants of both genders, belonging to different age groups.

## Clairvoyance

This is an esoteric tool for determining auric fields. clairvoyance or 'Clear sight' has been used for testing several healing modalities. More and more people are developing the ability to "see." While the ways in which people "see" often differ, the meanings are often remarkably similar. For example, symbols and colours, the energy activity and the size of the energy fields may all differ, however there is uniformity in interpretations of what they see.

The Pranic healers use clairvoyants to check for disease, blockages, malfunctions, etc., before a treatment and for the release of energy and changes in the disease state after a treatment. Everything that is done with the Pranic technique is evaluated clairvoyantly.

## Kirlian Photography

This is a method of photographing the electromagnetic field or aura that surrounds any living thing. This method was developed by two Russian scientists in the 1930's.

Professional Kirlian photographers say that they can easily recognize a Reiki healer because their auric field would always be much larger and more uniform than an average person.

There is another method of photography called "Aure Photographs," though it it is not scientifically valid. Therefore it should not be considered in the same class as Kirlian Photography.

## Dowsing

Dowsing is an ancient technique of discerning energy fields. Dowsing is probably best known because of its usefulness in locating water, usually in farming areas. These days dowsing is used to determine "Ley Lines" (an English term for energy fields present within the earth), electromagnetic fields (EMFs), and pathogenic fields of energy for buildings and land. Dowsing is also used to determine the auric fields of a person and complications related to it, appropriate diet, vitamins Homeopathic remedies, etc., and for communicating with your higher self for spiritual guidance.

Dowsing technique is very simple, hence it can be learnt quite easily. It may take you quite some time, however, to develop a high level of confidence in your answers. There are two primary methods of dowsing;

(1) RODS— **"L"** rods, or **"Y"** rods.

(2) PENDULUM— This can be anything hanging from a chain or string.

In case of dowsing with **"L"** Rods to measure the auric field both before and after Reiki treatments or attunements, it has been consistently found that there was an extensive increase in the size of the aura. As an example, on several occasions different people dowsed auric field of a Reiki Master while he was teaching and have found his auric field to be between 40 and 60 feet in radius, compared to a daily reading that used to be between 1 and 5 feet.

Pendulum is used to measure the length of the beam of energy coming from the hand chakra and fingertips both before and after Reiki attunements. The change in the force of the pendulum swing will be quite surprising.

# WORDS IN REIKI

**ACUTE:** Severe, but having short duration.

**ASTRAL BODY:** One of the subtle bodies just one frequency higher than the etheric body, also closely linked to the emotions; ethereal counterpart of body.

**AURA:** A subtle, invisible essence that emanates from humans, animals and other bodies; subtle emanation.

**ATTUNEMENTS:** Special Reiki initiations which raise the vibratory rate of the body, and open particular healing channels in the chakras.

**BIOPLASMIC BODY:** The Russian term for the L-field or etheric body

**BIOENERGETIC EXERCISES:** These are designed to generate electromagnetic energy in the body in order to move and release blockage.

**CHANNEL** (noun): The person who has emptied oneself to allow an alternate form of consciousness to flow through him.

**CHANNEL** (verb): To act as a human vehicle for the receiving and sending of information from any aspect of the All-Mind —spirit guide, own higher self, etc.).

**CHRONIC:** Lasting a long time.

**CRYSTAL GRIDWORK:** A geometric layout of crystals which is used to amplify healing and meditation.

**CENTER:** The point to place one's consciousness in the hara or belly chakra, to release the intellect and be at one with the All-Mind.

**CHAKRAS:** The energy centers located in the etheric body. They are closely linked to the endocrine system of the physical body.

**CAUSAL FACTOR:** Relates to the cause of disease—also the divine law of cause and effect. The causal body itself is one of the subtly bodies which stores all of our experiences.

**DISEASE:** Unhealthy condition of body, mind, plant, or some part thereof, illness, sickness; particular kind of this with special symptoms or location.

**ETHERIC BODY:** Bioplasmic body or energetic counterpart of the physical body, known as the L-field also.

**EXORCISM:** A ritual performed on the people who are thought to be possessed by evil spirits to drive the spirits out.

**ELEMENTALS:** These are repetitive thought forms which have taken on a life force of their own. Elementals can be seen by psychics in many different sizes and shapes.

**ENERGY BLOCK:** Refers to a point in both the etheric and physical bodies where energy has accumulated and cannot flow, due to disharmony or blockage in the body.

**HEALING:** A change which helps restore health.

**KIRLIAN PHOTOGRAPHY:** A special process developed to record on film the corona discharge, or aura, of the subject.

**L-FIELD:** The etheric or bioplasmic body.

**PLASMATIC STREAMING:** Release of energy through the system when an energy block is unclogged.

**PROCESS (to)** (verb): To digest or integrate therapy or information.

**PSYCHIC HEALING:** Healing which is performed through the projection of vibrations or energy, often from a distance.

**PSYCYCHIC SURGERY:** A form of psychic healing which focuses on the adjustment of the etheric body for healing purposes, and often has an outward appearance like actual surgery.

**PATTERNS (old behaviour):** Behaviour caused by habit, and often initiated by certain reactions to situations in the individual's past history.

**PHYSICAL CHEMICALIZATION:** The final release of toxins which cause disease. Mostly it causes a healing crisis in both acute and chronic cases.

**SUBTLE BODY:** The invisible (to normal eyesight) energy bodies (etheric, causal, and astral) of a higher vibratory frequency than the physical body.

**VIBRATORY LEVEL:** Refers to the various frequencies at which energy moves to and fro between two points.

## REIKI ORGANIZATIONS

**REIKI ALLIANCE**
P.O. Box 41, Cataldo ID 83810, 208/682-3535

**TRADITIONAL REIKI NETWORK**
FIRE No. 602 Case Hill Road, Treadwell NY 13846-0262
Tel & Fax : (607)829-3702
or
27, BETHLEHEM ROAD 93553 JERUSALEM, ISRAEL
Tel : 972-2-671-4964

**REIKI CENTER FOR HEALING ARTS**
SAN MATEO CA (415) 345-7666

**THE CENTER FOR REIKI TRAINING**
29209 North-Western Hwy # 592, Southfield MI 48034
Tel : (313) 948-8112

**BODHIDHARMA SCHOOL OF REIKI HEALING**
P.O. Box, 773, Avila Beach CA 93424

**REIKI OUTREACH INTERNATIONAL**
WORLD HQ : P.O. Box 609, Fair Oaks CA 95628, USA
Tel : (916)8-3-1500 Fax : (916) 863-6464
European Centre : P.O. Box 326, D-83090 Bad Endorf, Germany
Tel/Fax : 08053-9242

**REIKI INDIA RESEARCH CENTRE**
16-17 BA EKOPA,
Gunsagar Nagar, Station Road,
Kalwa, Thane, Mumbai - 400605
Tel. : 5413406, 5348243, 5363525

## INDIAN HEALERS

- **Sukhdeepak Malvai**
  **487, Sector 37, Noida (Uttar Pradesh) - 201303**
  **Tel. : 576451**

- **Meera Kotak**
  **Bangalore (Karnataka)**
  **Tel. : 3344314**

- **R. Nalini**
  **Chennai (Tamil Nadu)**
  **Tel. : 4881304**

- **Dr. K. Murlidharan**
  **Calcutta (West Bengal)**
  **Tel. : 4640056**

- **Tejinder Singh**
  **Chandigarh (Punjab)**
  **Tel. : 661586**